Cosmetics : A Practical Manual
Third Edition

Cosmetics : A Practical Manual
Third Edition

Dr. Swarnlata Saraf

Professor & Director
University Institute of Pharmacy,
Pt. Ravishankar Shukla University,
Raipur, Chhattisgarh, 492010.

Dr. Shailendra Saraf

Professor
University Institute of Pharmacy,
Pt. Ravishankar Shukla University,
Raipur, Chhattisgarh, 492010.

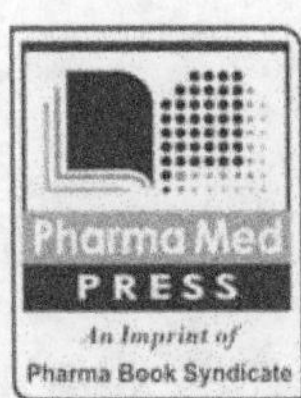

PharmaMed Press
An imprint of Pharma Book Syndicate

A unit of BSP Books Pvt. Ltd.

4-4-309/316, Giriraj Lane,
Sultan Bazar, Hyderabad - 500 095.

Published by

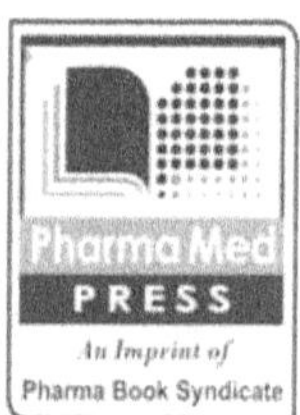

PharmaMed Press

An imprint of Pharma Book Syndicate

A unit of BSP Books Pvt. Ltd.

4-4-309/316, Giriraj Lane, Sultan Bazar, Hyderabad - 500095.
Phone: 040-23445605, 23445688; Fax: 91+40-23445611
E-mail: info@pharmamedpress.com

ISBN : 978-93-85433-62-7 (HB)

Preface to Third Edition

It is a matter of extreme pleasure for us that we are bringing back the revised edition of **"Cosmetics: A Practical Manual"**, with recent modifications and approaches that is according to the present need of the cosmetics.

World consumers are looking for personal care products that supply multiple benefits with minimal efforts. Their expectation lies in the latest technology advances that must be incorporated into innovative formulations. The trend governing the current therapeutic cosmetics has lead to a better understanding of modern ingredients and their assessment techniques. To obtain skin care formulations with real consumer-perceivable benefits and to optimize sensory attributes, formulators are resorting to these technologies. It is an era, in which not only women but males are also using cosmetics usually to enhance their own facial features. Cosmetics are products that are created for application on the body for the purpose of cleansing, beautifying or altering appearance and enhancing attractive features. Cosmetics are substances used to enhance the appearance or odour of the human body. Cosmetic pharmaceuticals, or cosmeceuticals, are cosmetic products that contain biologically active ingredients and claim to have medicinal or drug-like benefits.

In recent epoch, the herbal drug cosmaceuticals has brought drastic change in the field of conventional cosmetics. The mentality of herbal actives to be safe and effective has suddenly shifted the interest of consumers towards herbal drugs. As, a result, the herbal cosmetic industry is growing to and fro inspite of the recession in the economy. This can be proved by the report on the global market for anti-aging products and services which was worth $162.2 billion in 2008. This increased to $274.5 billion in 2013, with a compound annual growth rate (CAGR) of 11.1 percent. The boomers market has been the largest opportunity today in the world, mainly for their high disposable income. Therefore, all companies in the cosmetic, pharma and health care, biotech, medspa, and fitness services are strategizing hard to tap the double-digit growing boomer anti-aging market.

The most important botanicals pertaining to dermatologic uses such cosmaceuticals include teas, soy, pomagranate, date, grape seed, pycnogenol, horse chestnut, German chamomile, curcumin, allantoin, and aloe only green and black tea, soy, pomegranate, and date have been studied to the extent that clinical trials for the treatement of parameters of dermatological complications.

In addition to botanicals, other active compounds, such as enzymes, hyaluronic acid, amino acids, and peptides, also offering favorable opportunities in a variety of cosmaceutical products. Cosmeceutical development has also benefited the growth of other industries, such as nanotechnology. Keeping all these advancements in mind, we have revised the manual and done with some additions like herbal Anti-Ageing Preparations, Antioxidants, Herbal Cosmetics Containing Herbal Drugs, Skin Toners & Tonics, Herbal Sunscreens, Skin Depigmentating Agents which covers a broad area of expertization. It is for the first time that we are introducing a new informative chapter on "General Instruments For Cosmetics Evaluations" which will enable the student to be aware of the instruments used now-a-days in cosmetic labs. The revised edition also covers scientific description regarding the stability and toxicity of cosmetics in the chapters "Essentials of Stability Testing of Cosmetics" and "Assessment of Toxicity of Cosmaceuticals" respectively.

Thus, the approach and purpose of this book is to make aware the readers with different herbal based cosmaceuticals which are easy to prepare, based on their practical purpose. This book is an effort to enable the students with recent scenario of herbal cosmetics. It is an attempt to give category wise informations of herbal cosmetics in a very simple and informative way. The herbal formulas discussed in the relevant chapters comprises the knowledge regarding the type of raw materials used, nature and uses of the prepared formulation with ease of making the same.

We hope that the revised edition of this cosmetic manual will be highly informative, beneficial and will impart scientific understanding to the budding researchers at undergraduate level.

-Authors

Preface to First Edition

It gives us immense pleasure in bringing out the first edition of the book COSMETICS : A PRACTICAL MANUAL.

The approach and purpose of this book are different from those of the several excellent books on the formulation of dosage forms. No single book is available which covers the different practical aspects of cosmetics. This book informs the reader about the different types of practical cosmetic exercises or of the modern raw materials, however the major objective of this book is to serve as a practical manual for undergraduate students in the pharmaceutical sciences. The subject matter is presented in simple, concise and easily intelligible language. The salient features of the book are :

- The formulas and detailed methods of preparation of cosmetics have been included to help the students.
- The evaluation parameters are discussed separately.
- The properties of all the ingredients required for the cosmetic preparations are discussed with their safety and incompatibility parameters.

We have tried to make this book as informative and exhaustive as possible within the constraints of time allotted to the subject in the curriculum of different Universities. The efforts have also been made to incorporate the latest information available on the various cosmetic formulations to enable the students to accurately prepare various cosmetics in the laboratory.

We hope this book will be informative, beneficial and fulfill the demands of the undergraduate students of the Pharmacy.

-Authors

Contents

1

Introduction to Cosmetics

In 21st century, the winds of changes in the society are blowing forcefully in all parts of world for application of cosmetic. Cosmetic word is originated from Greek word "Kosmeticos" means adorn and preparation, which is used for this purpose, is known as cosmetic. We can define the cosmetic as "Cosmetic are external preparation meant for to apply on external part of the body i.e., nails, skin, hair for coloring, covering, softening, cleaning, nourishing, waving, setting, mollification, preservation, removal and protection" etc. We can also define it as "A cosmetic is an item intended to be rubbed, poured, sprinkled or sprayed on, introduced in to or otherwise applied to the human body or any part thereof for cleansing, beautifying, promoting attractiveness or altering the appearance".

All cosmetic preparation has their application for long or short periods to beautify the body as well as to keep the body healthy up to some extent and has psychological impact to other. The "active life" of any cosmetic preparation begins the moment it is brought in contact with the skin/hair/teeth/or nails and ends when it is removed or has evaporated. During it is active life; it has intimate reciprocal relationship, which results, cosmetic changes on the body. The cosmetic product prevents its outmost layer from drying out, penetrate below the external layer and introduce active substances in to deep lying strata or adhere only superficially to change color or luster of areas. The cosmetic which are used for decorative purposes, i.e., eye lines, rouges, mascara, face masking preparations etc and also carries the inherent risk of desirable side effects. It may inhibit important physiological process, chemically modify certain skin constituents (e.g., in case of bleaching and coloring preparations), and contribute towards their removal or even give rise to certain allergic reactions.

In modern cosmetology, the all products of cosmetic preparations manufactured under strict quality control conditions to achieve an absence of claims on both appearance and packing. There is varieties of cosmetic preparations are used which can be classifying by various ways :

(a) According to region, where it is use :

(i) *Skin :* Powder, Lipstick, Rouge, Creams, Lotions and Solutions etc.

(ii) *Hairs :* Shampoo, Conditioners, Creams, Bleach, Coloring preparation etc.

(iii) *Nails :* Nail lacquers, Lacquers removers etc.

(iv) *Teeth :* Powder, Paste, Gel and Dentifrices etc.

(v) *Eye :* Eyeliner, Mascara, Eye shadow and Eyebrow pencil etc.

(b) According to function of cosmetic preparation :

(i) *Emollient Preparation :* Cold creams, Vanishing creams, Foundation creams, Lotions and Solutions etc.

(ii) *Cleansing Preparation :* Creams, Shampoo and Rinses etc.

(iii) *Decorative Preparations :* Lipsticks, Rouges, Eyeliner, lacquers and Dressing preparations.

(iv) *Deodorant / Antiperspirant :* Spray, Sticks and Mouthwashes.

(v) *Protective Preparations :* Creams and Powders.

(vi) *Preparation for Enjoyment :* Salts, Powders, Oils and Milks.

(c) According to composition of cosmetics :

(i) Powder

(ii) Lotions

(iii) Emulsions

(iv) Solutions

(v) Suspensions

(vi) Creams

(vii) Paste

(viii) Gels

(ix) Aerosol

(x) Sticks

(xi) Pencils

A wide variety of cosmetics are available in the market. So, therefore, the knowledge of various cosmetics and their relative applications are given in this book.

Face Packs

Face packs are the preparations, which apply topically to facial area having high affinity to keratin and remain on skin surface. It is used for the purpose of achieving tightening sensation and a cleaning effect in the area of application. It adheres to skin surface and easily rubbed off. These are high viscosity or paste forms exemplified by the "Clay facial packs" and once fashionable "Mud packs". In general, they contain colloidal clay, kaolin or other suitable solids dispersed in a liquid vehicle. The desired plasticity is determined by concentration of solids.

The preparation is applied on facial area in lay thin film, 1/16" thick depth and allows remaining undisturbed until the evaporation of the water is substantially complete such evaporation may be hastened by forced ventilation. The loss of water causes the packs to harden and contract. The desired cleaning effect is due both the adsorptive efficiency of bentonite and to the process of removing the hardened pack. Regarding the removal of packs, it should prevent a complete dehydration of pack film should consist of humectants i.e. glycerol, to maintain plasticity of film sulfonated oils are used which also enhances cleaning efficiency.

There are other materials used in packs, for example, Alumina, Fuller's earth, Bone carcall and Kieselghur for its cleaning activity by adsorptive efficiency. Soluble colors are used to tint preparations as well to provide esthetic shades.

Now a day, in the formulation of "cleaning packs" special attention is paid to the inclusion of slightly abrasive ingredients in non-drying vehicle. The user applies the product by gentle massaging it into the skin after which is allowed to remain for a 10 – 20 minutes period. It is then removed, with the aid of a moistened towel. The ingredient used in such type of preparations are grain meals offering a wide latitude in particle size as well as intrinsic hardness, opacifier like Zinc Oxide, Titanic Dioxide and other metals like filtered honey crushed almond and preservatives.

Face Mask

Face Mask is the preparations, which are used to mask the skin imperfection and shininess. The skin imperfection are mainly red, rose, red spots, freckles, small birth marks, enlarged follicle mouth, scars of pervious skin lesions, wrinkles, exceptionally developed sebaceous and sweat gland etc. which can be mask by such type of preparations. These preparations generally have low viscosity and easily poured from the containers. All well formulated products should have some of the characteristics as follows:

1. It should produce allow ease of application and removal.
2. It should achieve their result without requiring under time drying.

3. It should be non-sensitizing and non-irritating to normal skin.

4. It should give superficial and mechanical effect to skin

Liquid mask are usually formulated around the film forming characteristics of one or more of the hydrophilic colloids like clay type components. They also have very satisfactory cleaning action by the inclusion of a small very satisfactory cleaning action by the inclusion of a small amount of mild but effective detergent. The masking effect is achieved with face powders, foundation creams and liquid make-ups and as auxiliary, day creams. Such type of preparation mainly covers the skin by a thin invisible film on the facial area. These preparations include basic powder material with adherent like opacifiers, colors and perfumes to provide smooth and shiny film.

Cold Cream

Historically the "Cold Cream" was known as "Ungerentum" or "Ceretum Refrigerence". Cold creams system is first reported by Galleon. It is water in oil type emulsion system with borax – bees wax combination as emulsifier. A protective film remains on skin following evaporation of water. The slow evaporation of water gives a skin cooling effect, so that it called "Cold Creams". These are used for cleaning, moisturizing, protective and also as sun screen creams. Cold creams become harder and more lustrous, the more oil it contains; with more water, it becomes softer. If it contains more than 60% of mineral oil it tends to bleed vegetable oils, occasionally make the creams granular. A smooth consistency of cold creams can be achieved by reducing warm component or adding lanolin or absorption base. It contains 10 – 20% of wax and above it, cream become ductile and salve like; spermaceti, kerosene and paraffin wax make it gloss where as lanolin provides softness. High melting waxes may provide bleeding of water during cooling process.

During the manufacturing of cold cream, temperature should be controlled to prevent discoloration, granule formation and bleeding of oil or water. Most commonly used perfume in cold cream is 'Rose', because it masks the fatty odor and no irritation effect. Cold cream frequently is referred to as a mixed emulsion, since oil in water as well as water in oil globules are present. Officially the cold cream is listed in United State Pharmacopoeia e.g., Rose water in USP and in NF XII.

Vanishing Creams

Vanishing creams are so termed because upon application and rubbing in to the skin, there is little or no visible evidence of their former presence. It forms a thin invisible film on skin followed by evaporation of water resulting non-glossy appearance. The basic nature of vanishing cream is oil in water emulsions, which are water removable because it contains o/w emulsifier. There two types of vanishing creams are available in markets; one is light vanishing cream, which have low binding capacity to powders and other heavy vanishing creams, which have strong capacity to bind with powders. Heavy vanishing creams are known as foundation creams, which are used as skin care product.

Cleansing Creams

Keeping the body clean is the first and most primitive demand on personal hygiene. The healthy body participates in the cleansing process just as it does in protecting itself against external disturbances. The cleansing creams remove visible soil from skin, hair and nails and dried perspiration's or removals of cosmetic preparations that makes the hair and skin sticky. The surface impurities of skin penetrate the corneal layer to some extent, that is removed by the skin in constant strengthening of the uppermost horney cells and rubbed off by normal activities of the body. The skin resident flora also assists in the degradation and removal of organic impurities. But such type of cleaning is not enough as cosmetic point of views, so we use the cleansing preparations like creams and lotions.

The cleansing preparation contains mainly soap with other adjustments like SAA, solubilizing agents, swelling agents, absorbents. There are two types of cleaning preparations are available in markets. One is water based skin cleansing and another is oil-based skin cleansing preparation. The mechanism of skin cleansing is mainly by dispersing the surface foreign materials in oil and water emulsion and then rinse off by several washings without water. Oily creams solubilize the foreign particles and some of the cleansing creams absorb the surface soil then rinse off with water.

After Shave Lotions

After-shave lotions relieve the feeling of tautness and discomfort caused by shaving. It is use to refresh, cool the skin, smooth miner irritations and impart the feeling of well being. There are varieties of after-shave lotions available in market, i.e., clear lotions, stick lotions and gels, creams and emulsified lotions. Some other types of after-shave preparations also available like powders, pencils, alum blocks and aerosols etc. Such formulations have one or more special characteristics, which dictate the physical form of the product and relative efficiency when used after different types of shaves.

Fragrance feels continue to be primary considerations in the formulation of after-shave. Its formulation also consider mild astringency, neutralization of soap left on skin to help restore normal acid mantle and anti bacterial action. Most of the after-shave lotions contain 40 to 60% by volume of alcohol for cooling mild astringency and refreshing. Emolliency is imparted readily by use of humectants (up to 3% of polyols). The antiseptics are usually employed at concentration below 0.1% of active ingredients such as quaternary compounds and phenols. After-shave creams and emulsified lotions are also utilized by men, who find an alcoholic after-shave lotion dis-comfortable i.e., irritation in wind, sun and inclement weather. These emulsified lotions are simply emollient vanishing cream or hard lotions to furnish off the shave. "Witch hazelifiam" or "Snow" is examples of after-shave emulsified lotions.

Shampoo

Shampoo can be defined as a preparation of a surfactant in suitable form liquid, solid or powder. Which when used under the condition specified will remove surface grease, dirt and skin debris from hair shaft and scalp without affecting adversely the hair, scalp or health of the user. Shampoo leave the hair fragrant soft, lustrous and manageable. The formulation of a shampoo should have special capabilities like minimizing eye sting, controlling dandruff or imparting appealing fragrance to gain more favorable acceptance from particular segments of the population. There are variety of forms and types of shampoos are available in the market due to its unusual compensate and their combination such as;

  (i)   Children's and infants shampoo.

  (ii)   Shampoo for dry, oily and normal hairs.

  (iii) Shampoo for men etc.

The most common form of the shampoo is cream and gel shampoos because of its high stability during storage and good efficiency. There are varieties of forms are available in the market like liquid, cream, gel, powder and aerosol etc. The major component of the shampoo is surfactant (soaps and synthetic detergent) with other additions like conditioners, sequestering agents, rinsing components (acids), foam builders, opacifying agents, clarifying agents (e.g. EDTA) anti-dandruff agent, thickening agent, preservatives, stability additives and other cosmetic additions (e.g. perfume and dyes). The special variety of shampoo is also available.

  (a) ***Acid Balanced Shampoo :*** As the term "acid balanced shampoo" called the balance of acidic nature of fatty acids of oils used in shampoo to maintain the "acid mantle of skin". This is achieved by optimum concentration of alkaline compounds in shampoo.

  (b) ***Egg Shampoo :*** The Egg Shampoo is a type of special shampoo where shampoo is used as base and egg is for its special material to contact with the hair. Egg shampoo is used for its conditioning, nourishing as well as cheer effect to the hairs.

Talcum Powders

Talcum powders are the protective preparations against mechanical stress, which act as skin lubricants and cooling agent. Minute particles of powder have large surface area results in strong light dispersion, which visually covers the skin underneath. The surface of powdered skin exposed to air is much larger than that of un-powdered skin, so it leads to cooling effect. The fine particles and its lightweight, powder adheres to the skin by stickiness of the fat film and relief the skin from gravity and rubbing to remove it. The talcum powder consists of talc as main ingredients with additives like absorbent, adherent, covering agent, perfumes, heat conducive agents, fragrance and antioxidants etc.

Face Powder

A face powder is basically a cosmetic product, which has as its prime functions the ability to complement skin color by imparting velvet like finish. It enhances the appearance of the skin by masking the shine due to the secretion of sebaceous and sweats glands. Powder achieve its effect by being opaque enough to mask minor blemishes, but not import a mask like effect, It posses reasonably lasting properties. So that re-powdering frequently is unnecessary. It consists of various constituents, which imparts essential characteristics of a good product: -

1. *Covering Powder :* The ability to mask skin defects such as skin shine, enlarge pores and minor blemishes, e.g., zinc oxide, titanium dioxide etc.

2. *Slip :* The degree of spreading over the skin without dragging, and giving the characteristic smooth feeling, e.g., talc, aluminum hydrosillicate, zinc and magnesium soaps of higher fatty acids etc.

3. *Adhesiveness :* The ability to cleaning to the face e.g., zinc and magnesium stearates etc.

4. *Absorbency :* The capacity of absorbing skin secretions (perspiration and oiliness) without showing evidence of such absorption, e.g., colloidal kaolin, magnesium and calcium carbonate etc.

5. *Bloom :* The ability to impart a velvety, peach like finish to the skin, e.g., starches, guanine and bismuth chloride.

Compact Powder

Compact powder is a type of face powder compressed in to a cake and applied with a powder puff. It is more popular because of its ease in application, storage and convenience. Its formulation is same as face powder except it contains more concentration of binders. It has larger particle size than normal face powder and more adherences to the skin. It contains basic face powder ingredients like covering power agents, slipping agents, bloom and peach finish agent, absorbent, adherent, coloring agent and binding agent with preservatives.

There are varieties of binding agents like dry binder, oil binder, water-soluble or water repellant and emulsion binders are mostly used in compact. Because of the presence of binder, which are mostly susceptible to microbial attack, so most useful preservatives like p-hydroxy benzoate is used in formulation. Compacts are manufactured by various methods, such as wet method, dry method and damp method. Most commercially useful method is damp method.

Tooth Powder

Tooth powder is a preparation used for cleaning as well as therapeutic dentifrices. Most commonly its formulation consist of calcium carbonate as polishing agent, sodium soap like sodium lauryl sulfate as surface-active agent, mixture of insoluble sodium metaphosphate and tricalcium phosphate as an abrasive. Variety of the tooth powders available in the market according to their active constituents like ammoniated tooth powders, chlorophyll tooth powders, penicillin tooth powder and fluoride tooth powder etc. Tooth powder manufacturing consists of a homogeneous mixing of all ingredients without contamination of foreign solutions either added.

Tooth Paste

Toothpastes are the preparation intended for use with a toothbrush for the purpose of cleaning the accessible surface of the teeth. It enhance personal appearance by maintaining cleaner teeth, brushing with it reduce the tooth decay, helps to maintain healthy gingival and reduces the intensity of mouth odors. There are varieties of toothpaste are available in the market according to their components proposed for use in. Therapeutic purpose like chlorophyll toothpaste to prevent gingival disease and carries; anti-enzyme tooth paste for preventing dental carries; fluoride tooth paste for giving hardness and lasting quality to tooth structure and as anti-dental carries and cleaning purpose like ammoniated toothpaste loose the dental plaque by chemical reaction and make them susceptible to removal by tooth brushing.

The general formulation of toothpaste contains various ingredients for their special properties are as follows: -

1. *Abrasives :* It removes debris; residual stains from teeth and polishing agent. The agents uses for this purpose are calcium carbonate, dibasic calcium phosphate dehydrate, tricalcium phosphate, insoluble sodium metaphosphate, hydrated alumnae and calcium pyrophosphate etc.

2. *Surface-active agents :* These agents lower surface tension to improving cleaning and also for foaming characteristics, e.g., sodium lauryl sulphate, sodium coconut monoglyceride sulfanate and sodium N-lauryl sarcosinate etc.

3. *Humectants :* It is used to retain moisture or prevent paste from hardening of paste when it expose to air, e.g., glycerol, sorbitol and propylene glycol etc.

4. *Binders :* These are used to prevent separation of liquid phase from solid, particularly during storage, e.g., glycerite of starch, natural tree exudates, seaweed colloids, like Iris moss alginates and veegum etc.

5. *Flavors :* These are used to impart taste of paste. Most command flavors used in pastes are spearmint, peppermint, wintergreen and cinnamon-mint etc.

6. *Miscellaneous :* Therapeutics Ingredients like chlorophyll, fluorides, anti-enzymes agent and antibiotic etc.

Denture Cleaners

Dentures are similar to material teeth, which may develop plaques, deposits of tartar and brown spots due to smoking. So its cleaning is necessary to prevent an inflammation of gingival underneath. Denture cleaners are always available in the market are dry powders or tablets. They remain dry till they are used otherwise it become unattractive and loss their effectiveness. These are quickly dissolved in water to give clear solution. These preparations often contain common salt which act as filler and promotes the precipitation and removal of proteins in impurities. Alkaline salts such as trisodium phosphate and sodium carbonate etc., supports the action of surface-active agents. Denture cleaners usually consist of following substances or groups of sustainers.

1. Chemical active substances that degrade plaque and tartar, e.g., sodium hypochloride, sodium perborate and urea peroxide.

2. Surfactant facilitating the wetting of the denture and impurities on it.

3. Disinfectant.

4. Flavors, which mainly used in paste formulation.

5. Dyes to enhance esthetic appeal.

6. The use of denture cleaners are very simple just by placing denture over night or for 30 minutes in denture cleaning solution and then wash off with water.

Hair Conditioners

Hair conditioners are the preparations, which maintain the condition of hairs. Almost every hair preparations are claimed to hair conditioners. The products which involve with the mechanical and surface properties of hair like lubricity, manageability, substantively and sheen are enter in to hair conditioning can be achieved by various ways.

1. The products maintain the conditioning by improving ordering of cuticle scales resulting smooth hair surface, such type of products are simple acidic rinses.

2. The products, which adsorb chemical compounds in to the cuticle of hair resulting sheen, gloss and lubricity, such type of compounds, are Lewis acids and SAA.

3. The products containing proteins, such as collagen derived pepticles, (i.e., casein, albumin) which act optimum at pH 6.0 and absorb in to the damaged hair shaft to maintain conditions of hair.

4. The product-containing surface achieves agent, which act as ceroplastic and substantive to hair. It absorb by damaged hair to maintain its electrostatic nature, e.g. tetra alkyl substituted amine salt.

5. The oils and waxes containing product lubricate the hair shaft and improve optical properties of hairs, e.g. Brilliantine, cholesterol, lanolin, silicone oil and panthenal etc.

Lipsticks

Lipstick is generally accepted essential and leading makeup device available in variety of luster and texture. It is composed essentially of a oil-wax base, stift enough to form a stick with a staining dye dissolved or dispersed in the oil, and pigment suspended there in, suitable perfumed and flavored, molded and enclosed in a case. The lipstick provides a convenient means of freshening the make-up. Lipsticks impart attractive color, glossy and most appearance to lips, accentuating good points and distinguishing the defects. The properly applied lipstick totally changes the apparent facial appearance. It also prevents cracking and chafing of lips to lead bacterial infection. It also provides emollient action to the lips. The formulation of lipsticks consists of oil and wax mixture having desired melting point and viscosity. The range of melting point choose for this mixture is 55°C to 75°C and most commonly used is 62°C for hot climatic areas. It also contains bromo mixture to impart indelible stain and colors or pigments. The other ingredients, which are used in lipstick formulation, are preservatives, fragrance, surfactant and stabilizers, emulsifiers and antioxidants etc.

Eye Liners

It is the oldest and most extensively used cosmetics for enhancing the eyes. It is a preparation, which harmonized with shades of mascara. Originally it is liquid dispersion but now as the development proceeds, it is successfully replaced by emulsified product, i.e. cream or cake. This preparation is formulated in such a way that can applied in a thin line cannot cake and water-resistant. Now a day, shiny and matte **eyeliners** are available in the market. These various types of eyeliners are available, i.e. lustrous, liquid eyeliner, cake or frosted cake eyeliner etc. The formulation of eyeliner consists of pigments or dyes, waxes, oils, gums, esters, preservatives, pearle scent and perfumes etc. High shine eyeliner is made by using material as latex (cosmetically safe) or carboset with addition of plasticizer such as glycerol, polyvinyl alcohol and polyvinyl acetate etc. The coloring agent which are most commonly used are carbon black, iron and chromium oxide pigments, carmine NF, and cochineal etc., which are FDA certified pigments. To achieve lighter and pastel shades titanium dioxide or zinc oxide is employed with pigments.

Liquid Soaps

Liquid soaps are generally defined as aqueous solutions of the salts of fatty acids. Originally they are obtained by saponifying the natural animal and vegetable fats and oils with alkali, as sodium and potassium hydroxide. But now alkyl amines are used as alkali, e.g., triethanolamine is most commonly used. It forms stable foam and less strong alkali reaction than sodium and potassium alkali. Production of good liquid soap by total saponification of neutral fats is an art, which require much experience. The soaps prepared from fatty acids with fever than 10 carbons (coconut oil, palm oil and castor oil etc.) in the chain gives too soluble soap to form acceptable suds or to show acceptable detergency. Where as the soaps of fatty acids with more than 20 carbons are too insoluble to function effectively at normal temperature. Commonly used soaps have pH range from 7 – 10.

The soap solution having pH10 - cause solubilization of skin lipids and cause dryness but the nearly neutral pH having soap solutions does not cause any harmful effect. Now a days, super fatted soap solutions are used which have lower pH in aqueous solution with emollient effect on skin. Most commonly used cleaning agent in liquid soap is sodium coconut fatty acids isethionate for dry and scaly skin. Others cleaning agents used, as detergent emulsion are sodium alkylphenoxy polyether sulfonate and alkyl ethanol imidazolinium sodium carbonate with other additives such cholesterol, petrolatum and perfumes. The advantages of these agents provide good cleaning with stable foaming properties. Some examples of marketed liquid soaps are Dettol Soap, Lifebuoy's liquid soap etc.

Baby Powders

The skin of babies is differing from adult both in histological and physiologically. It is thinner, less cornified and less hairy. It contains higher proportion of water and extra-cellular fluid material lacking in classic reticulum in structure. The baby powders are used principally as lubricant in skin folds to prevent chafing, to absorb perspiration, as water repellant to relieve prickly heat, to impart cleanliness and for pleasant fragrance to baby's skin.

The baby powder composition is similar to ordinary powder composition is similar to ordinary powder except it contain antiseptics, not highly perfumed flat, rounded and platelets shape. The best size of particle is 325 or 44 um range. Talc and natural hydrous magnesium silicate is the most important constituent of baby powders because it has excellent slip characteristics and good adhesion to the skin. Commonly raw-materials used for baby powder formulations are lithium stearate as adherent, olive oil to improve adherence and emollience, zinc oxide as opacifier to burning rays of the sun, astringent, neutralizing power soothing effect, colloidal kaolin to control power bulk property, unduecyclinates as antifungal and anti-bacterial agent, mild perfumes and boric acid as antiseptic etc. .

Packing of Cosmetics

The container should be selected carefully for cosmetic packaging to ensure that there is no interaction between cosmetic ingredient and packaging material. It must be ascertain that neither odour development due to glues nor any incompatibility between material of container and product being employed. The packaging operation plays an important role in stated parameters on the container. The packaging materials, which are commonly used, are plastic (PVC and PE) bottles and tubes for toiletries. Shampoos rinsed and liquid cosmetics are packed in containers having good barrier properties for water vapor, essential oils and air through container pores. Paste and solid cosmetics are package in metal like tin, aluminum, lead and most preferably plastic containers. Metal containers if used then they are coated internally by polyethylene or wax lining or dentifrices to protect corrosion. Dentifrice contains collapsible tubes, which is laminated structure comprising aluminum foil, layers of paper and polyethylene with plastic nozzle. Aluminum tube should not be used for fluoride containing paste. Fluoride containing paste is package in lead tube, which is internally coated with wax. Powders are mostly pack in tin plated or chemically treated steel or internally coated with suitable lacquer.

2

Evaluation of Cosmetics

The cosmetics are evaluated for its performance, efficiency, storage, processing operations and its stability approved. There are variety of parameters are used for the evaluations.

Evaluation of Facial Cosmetics

There are variety of facial preparations are used in cosmetics, such as face powder, compact powder and talcum powder. These preparations are evaluated for their quality control analysis and finally for its effectiveness. The facial preparation is a mixture of many ingredients. Which contribute to its desired properties: covering power, slip, adhesiveness, absorbency, perfume, color, bloom and bulking. These properties can be evaluated by the following parameters.

(a) *Physical Parameters*

(i) *Color :* The color of powder should be nearly skin tone to provide covering of blemishes of skin, without its visibility.

(ii) *pH :* The 1-gram of product with 9 gram of water and shake vigorously then determine pH by glass or low range pH paper in aqueous solution.

(iii) *Adhesiveness :* It is a characteristic of particle size and shape and checked by simply rubbing the powder on skin. If no any eruptions and rashes, then consider as free from grittiness.

(iv) *Net content :* Place the opened can with the frozen material in a beaker and warm it to room temperature. Decant the content and weigh the container, calculate the content by difference.

(v) *Odor :* By smelling the product.

(vi) *Size and shape of particle :* Spread a pinch of powder on a slide in to a thin layer and observe under microscope with the help of micrometers (size), size of particles can be evaluated by sieve analysis method.

(vii) *Moisture content :* Moisture content is tested by any analytical method, such as titrimetric method.

2. Esthetic Evaluation

(i) *Shade Control :* This evaluation is mostly carried out in face powder and compact powders to control production that should not be differ to any appreciable degree from standard batches under normal light. It can be evaluated by two ways: -

(a) Spread out powder on a white paper and in back ground, having skin tone color. Then it is compare in appearance to skin tone, which is used as a standard.

(b) Sample color is compare to the standard by skin tone (undertone).

If in both testing if color shading is similar to skin tone, then it ultimately result consumers method of evaluation and usage.

(ii) *Dispersion of Color :* This evaluation is done for checking uniform distribution of colors and pigments in powder to check color streaks or incompatibility in powder dispersion due to poor pulverization or bleeding of color. Spreading the powder on white paper and examining with magnifying glass can carry it out. If any un-uniformity is observed the batch is further process for homogeneity.

(iii) *Bloom Testing :* It is tested by with the help of photo Val photometer or polarizing filter after spreading a thin layer of powder on white paper then compare to normal skin.

Test for adhesiveness to skin or pay off:

(iv) *Testing :* The pay off property of powder provides adherence power of powder to skin. It is always be checked on skin. A puff applied on cake or powder with little pressure then it is rub on the skin. If complete attached powder to puff is pay off on skin, then powder is considered a good pay off quality. This pay off quality is also dependent on degree of hardness of the powder.

(v) *Test for handling or Breaking Test :* This test is also applicable for compact powder to predict handling powder. The test is performed by dropping the cake with packing from 8 to 10 inch heights on a wooden surface several times. If cake remains unbroken, then it is an indication of normal handling of powder without unsatisfactory results.

(vi) *Spreadability :* It is tested by angle of repose, it is comes under the value of 30° then, powder is considered as good spreadability power.

(vii) *Covering Power :* A pinch of powder with the help of puff is applied on skin, if it is completely mask the skin without showing clowny appearance then it is consider as good covering power.

3. **Testing of process of manufacturing or pressure testing :** This evaluation is specially applied for compacts for checking the presence of air pockets in cakes. If any air pockets in cakes then compact can easily be broken by little pressure. This testing is carried out by the help of penetrometer, in which uniform pressure is applied on cake and reading of proper hardness result absence of air pockets.

4. **Evaluation of Dentifrices :** Abrasiveness Testing: Brush the teeth with dentifrices for 10 minutes then enamel is used as testing surface for abrasion. If negligible rash observed on enamel surface, then dentifrices considered as good.

   (i) *Determination of degree of luster production :* It is evaluated by light reflection, which is measured by photometer or photo filter and compare to standard.

   (ii) *Consistency:* It is applicable for paste and denture cleaners.

   (iii) *Specific Gravity :* Specifically carried out for powder to select container capacity.

   (iv) *pH :* Tested by dissolving 1 gram product in to 9 gram of water shake vigorously then aqueous solution pH is observed by pH meter.

   (v) *Odor, Taste and Color :* Tested simply observation by smack and visually.

   (vi) *Moisture Content :* It is checked in paste cleaners for indication to prevent hardening of paste, when exposed to air checked by titrimetric method.

   (vii) *Fragrance Test :* By individually observation for its acceptability.

Evaluation of Hair Conditioners

Evaluation of hair conditioning is basically dependent on subjective appraisal. The degree of conditioning is judged by users past experience, present experience and a continuing change in the individual scalp and hair situation.

1. *Softness :* It is tested by various ways as follows: -
   (i) Softness is evaluated by a sense of resilience, smoothness of feel (handle) and a freedom for stickiness and stiffness.

(ii) It is evaluated by attendant reduction or elimination of snarls and tangling.

(iii) By measuring the electrostatic charge after conditioning the hair with the help of suitable apparatus.

2. *Luster :* The luster of hair is measure by degree of reflection of light with the help of photo volt photometer and a polarizing filter with comparison to standard value.

3. *Lubricity :* The lubricity test gives frictional aspect of hair, which depends on the outer surface, the cuticle. It is evaluated by an instrument for measuring dry hair respiness with an electronic comb, which measure friction during combing.

4. *Body, Texture and Set Retention :* This evaluation is completely depends on the individual evaluation ratings. The conditioning hairs if do not retain its set are termed as "limp" or "too fine" and set is retain (or strong adherence) then conditioner is termed "coarse" or wiry conditioner.

5. *Irritation and Toxicity :* Such test is performed for safety point of view to provide its acceptability.

(i) *Eye irritation test :* It is performed on rabbits mostly and some times monkeys are also use. Drip a drop on rabbit eye mucosa then count no of blinking in a period of time and this numbering is compare to normal blinking and tears. If no tearing and similar blinking to normal eye, then conditioner considers as good.

(ii) *Oral Toxicity Test :* It is evaluated on dog by measuring the LD/50 or Lethal dose, i.e. number of material per kg of body weight required to kill half of the test animal employed. If LD/50 is 5 or higher, then conditioner is considering as lower toxicity.

6. *Fragrance Test :* This test provides degree of acceptability by person and depends completely on consumer's appeal. It is evaluated by the following ways: The fragrance sniffed in the bottle.

(i) The fragrance encounters, users during practical use.

(ii) The radial fragrance left on the hair after rinsing, drying and coiffing.

(iii) The stability of fragrance during its storage.

In all ways if more than 100 subjects accept it then product is considered be good.

7. *Color :* Tested by simple visual observations after conditioning of hairs.

8. *Consistency :* It provides the fluidity of the product measured by Viscometer.

Evaluation of Herbal Cosmetics

The herbal cosmetics are to be evaluated for the following evaluations:

1. *Physical Evaluations*
   - (i)   Color
   - (ii)   Odor
   - (iii)   Form of Physical State
   - (iv)   pH : 10-dilution solution pH is measured by pH meter.
   - (v)   Net Content : Weigh the packed product then weigh without product. The difference of weight gives net content weight.
   - (vi)   Others- Ash examination, saponification values, and acid values were determined according to methods discussed by Lachman *et al*. 1992. Fatty content and nonvolatile content should be determined.

2. *Sensitivity Test* : It is tested by "Patch Test". Apply product on 1 cm^2 patch of skin, if no any inflammation or rashes then it considered as free from sensitivity.

3. *Irritation Test* : It is carried out by applying product on the skin for 10 minutes. If no irritation then it is considered as non-irritating product.

4. *Grittiness* : A pinch of product is rubbed on skin and then observed with magnifying glass; if its free from rashes or eruption then it is considered as free from grittiness.

Bleeding Test

Such type of evaluations is carried out for semi solid preparation. The products are kept frequently for a period of time alternatively in fridge and at room temperature then bleeding of liquid is observed, if no liquid phase is omit out then it is considered as stable product for climatic conditions.

Rheology

To study flow property of liquid or semi solid product, it is performed: -

- (i)   *Spreadability* : A pinch of product should be easily spreadable on skin.
- (ii)   *Pourability* :
  - (a)   The liquid product should be easily poured out from the bottle. The rate of coming out should not be too fast and nor be too slow. This effect will also provide retention period of cosmetic at skin.
  - (b)   If semi solid product is in container, then it should have thixotropic property.

Microbial Test

It is tested by microbial assay method as per specification given in Pharmacopoeia.

Diffusibility

It is evaluated by "Agar Cup Method" and degree of diffusibility is predicted by comparing with standard by calculating the diameter of product diffusion using suitable indicator in agar medium.

Toxicity Test

It is tested by lethal dose or LD/50 count.

Stability Studies

The stability studies are carried out at elevated temperature, relative humidity and pH environment by its physical observations regularly in 6 months of period.

Evaluation of Preservatives

1. *Thin layer chromatography*

   Thin layer chromatography can be used, as a rapid means of screening a cosmetic to identify which preservative is present.

2. *Partition chromatography*

   The following partition chromatographic method separates the preservative of interest from the remainder of the cosmetic by elution on a partition column of silanized Celite with various concentrations of acidified alcohol. The eluants are examined by UV spectrophotometery and the preservative is determined quantitatively.

3. *Formaldehyde and its releasers by fluorescence spectroscopy*

   Several preservatives that are difficult to identify can frequently be detected by conversion to a highly fluorescent derivative. In the method formaldehyde or a formaldehyde-releasing compound is condensed with acetyl acetone and ammonia in a buffered aqueous solution to give a highly fluorescent dihydrolutidine derivative whose concentration can be determined by measuring its fluorescence.

4. Pyrolysis

5. Digestion- aeration

6. Gas liquid chromatography

7. High pressure liquid chromatography

Efficacy Evaluation

Modern techniques are available to evaluate the efficacy of all cosmetic products (either synthetic or herbal). Various instruments are described below which\h are use for efficacy testing of cosmetic on skin.

Evaluation parameter		**Instruments used**
1.	Hydration/mositurizing effect	- Cutometer, Multimeter
2.	Skin firmness	- Cutometer
3.	Skin Elasticity	- Cutometer, Blastiometer
4.	Erythema	- Corneometer
5.	Sunscreen Protection Factor determination	- Solarimeter
6.	Skin glowness	- Luxameter
7.	Transdermal epidermal loss (TEWL)	- Tewameter, Mexameter
8.	Skin PH	- Skin pH meter
9.	Skin sebum	- Sebumeter
10.	Skin friction	- Skin Friction meter

3

Cosmetic Excipients

The term excipient comes from the Latin word excipients, present participle of the verb excipere, which means to receive, to gather, and to take out. This refers to one of the properties of an excipient, which is to ensure that a product has the weight, consistency and volume necessary for the correct administration of the active principle to the patient. In 1957, excipients were defined as 'the substance used as a medium for giving a active principals, that is to say with simply the functions of an inert support of the active principle or principles. Again, in 1974 they are described as 'any more or less inert substance added to a prescription in order to interpretation of the adverb 'intentionally' brings to mind the multiple roles that an excipient must play today in a modern pharmaceutical and cosmetic products, suitable to use topically.

Generally speaking, excipients account for most of the weight or volume of a product. In a world pharmaceutical and cosmetic market valued at about £ 215 billion, that of the excipients amounts to about £1.5 billion, 42% of which in North America, 33% in Europe and 25% in the rest of the world. In 1999, all this corresponded to 600 thousand tons of materials most of which for the food, cosmetic and chemical industries and only a small part for the pharmaceutical industry. Excipients are of various origins: animal (e.g. lactose, gelatin, stearic acid), plant (e.g. starches, sugars, cellulose, alginates), mineral (e.g. calcium phosphate, silica) and synthesis (e.g. PEGs, polysorbates, povidone, etc.) and they often lack a trade name. Their origin and use do not often guarantee the quality required by the industry, which must therefore submit them to more thorough-going analytical controls. In order to carry out the numerous functions required, new classes of excipients have now become available, derived from old and new materials, alone or in combination, adapted to the manufacture of high-performance products. Looking at the matter from this angle, excipients can no longer be considered mere inert supports for the active principles, but essential functional components of a modern formulation. The requirement of excipient in society is in developing stage as the growth of industrialization in the community. These are beneficial by introduction of synthetic materials hardly damage skin any more than old soap based preparation.

Ideal Characteristics of Cosmetic Excipients

The all excipients must meet certain criteria in the formulation. These include the following:

1. They must be non toxic and acceptable to the regulatory agencies in all countries where the cosmetic product is to be marketed.
2. They must be preventing skin from harmful effect.
3. They must be impenetrable to skin.
4. They should remain active for a reasonable time in preparation.
5. The properties of material must be such that- should not be easily rubbed or pealed of the skin.
6. They must be free of any unacceptable microbial load.
7. The materials should not form brittle film on the skin even under prolonged mechanical stress.
8. The material should be removable without too much scrubbing or use of strongly degreasing solvent (acetone, benzene etc.).
9. They must be physiologically inert.
10. Their cost must be acceptably low.
11. They should be easily applicable and pleasant to use.

Selection of Excipients

A vast range of cosmetic excipeints is available but their selection will depends on its physico-chemical properties and their compatibility to product. No one material possesses all the desired characteristics though some possess more than one attribute. Some criteria for the selection are discussed here:

1. The ingredients of cleansing creams and lotion, which may be emulsifier, detergents, antiseptics and solvents. The very in nature of the cleansing process itself dictate the selection of rational as per need e.g., adequate safety if mechanical rubbing is utilized for cleansing process.
2. The huge increase in the use of eye make-up has created a need for means of removal mineral oil or isopar, alone, is a safe, effective agent for the removal of eye make-up.

3. The emollients comprise a long list of materials in which mineral oil and petrolatum are frequently major component in cosmetic formulation, and their effects must be considered in as much as they are completely occlusive emollients.

4. In hormone creams a rigid quality control procedure must be applied with thorough standardization of raw materials and accurate assaying of the hormone.

5. The selection of raw materials for the baby toiletries should be preceded by patch testing of each ingredient separately.

6. Some people may be sensitive to skin lighteners and bleach creams so care should be taken during selection of excipients.

7. Oily vehicles tend to more effective for producing a uniform and long lasting film of sunscreen on the skin and their emollient properties protect the skin against the drying effect of exposure to wind and sun.

8. The primary consideration of choice of excipients in face powder is based on the type i.e., compact, loose powder and talcum powder etc. The basic ingredient used and its quality plays an important role in the ultimate powder formulation.

9. Dentifrice containing insoluble sodium metaphosphate as the abrasive was more effective in maintaining clean teeth than dentifrices containing chalk, tricalcium phosphate or dicalcium phosphate.

10. The conventional shaving soaps and lather shave creams seldom are lacking in beard- softening action, so modified excipients reformulate brush less shave cream to increase its beard- softening, moisturizing, skin lubricating and skin protecting properties.

11. Sulfide raw material in depilatory cosmetic preparation is utilized in quick hair removing preparation as compare to calcium thioglycolate containing preparation.

12. A shampoo formulation excipients selection based on some specialized capability like minimizing eye sting, controlling dandruff or imparting appealing fragrance to gain a more favorable acceptance.

13. The selection of raw materials in hair grooming preparation based on good grooming, luster without greasiness, protection from the elements and some degree of hair conditioning.

14. To improve the technology regarding art with suitable excipients related to the hair straightening process on own desire; the selection of raw material can play an important role.

15. Selection of excipients in hair conditioners, lacquers, setting lotions based on so many factors like product stability, proper methods of product preservation and the perfuming of the product must also be considered.

16. The selection of raw material for the dental restorations and in fingernail elongates based on ease of polymerization, its availability, toxicity and strength.

17. Choice of coloring preparations, preservatives and raw materials is limited to approval of FDA.

Talc

Talc is a purified, hydrated, magnesium silicate, approximating to the formula $Mg_6(Si_2O_5)_4(OH)_4$. It may contain small, variable amounts of aluminum silicate and iron.

Synonyms

Magsil Osmanthus; Magsil Star; Powdered talc; Purified french chalk; Purtalc; soapstone; Steatite.

Molecular Formula : $Mg_6(Si_2O_5)_4(OH)_4$.

Characteristics

Talc is a very fine, white to grayish-white colored, odorless, impalpable, unctuous, crystalline powder. It adheres readily to the skin, is soft to the touch, and free from grittiness.

Pharmaceutical Applications

Talc was once widely used in oral solid dosage formulations as a lubricant and diluents. It is not as common today. Also it is now being used as a dissolution retardant in the development of controlled-release products. As far as topical preparations it is used as a dusting powder, although it should not be used to dust surgical gloves. Since talc is a natural material it may frequently contain microorganisms and should therefore be sterilized when used as a dusting powder.

Talc is additionally used to clarify liquids and is also used, mainly for its lubricant properties, in cosmetics and food products.

Stability and Storage Conditions

Talc is a stable material and may be sterilized by heating at 160°C for not less than 1 hour. It may also be sterilized by exposure to ethylene oxide or gamma irradiation. Talc should be stored in a well-closed container in a cool and dry place.

Incompatibilities

Incompatible with quaternary ammonium compounds

Glycerin

Nonproprietary Names : BP: Glycerol, JP: Concentrated Glycerin, PhEur: Glycerolum

USP : Glycerin

Synonyms

Croderol; E422; glycerine; Glycon G-100; Kemstrene; Pricerine; 1,2,3-propanetriol; Trihydroxypropane glycerol.

Molecular Formula

$C_3H_8O_3$ (92.09)

Pharmaceutical Applications

Glycerin is used in a wide variety of pharmaceutical formulations including oral, otic, ophthalmic, topical, and parenteral preparations. It is also used in cosmetics and as a food additive. In topical pharmaceutical formulations and cosmetics, glycerin is used primarily for its humectants and emollient properties. In parenteral formulations glycerin is mainly used as a solvent. In oral solutions glycerin is used as a solvent, sweetening agent, antimicrobial preservative, and viscosity- increasing agent. Glycerin is also used as a plasticizer of gelatin in the production of soft-gelatin capsules and gelatin suppositories. Glycerin is additionally employed as a therapeutic agent in a variety of clinical applications.

Stability and Storage Conditions

Glycerin is hygroscopic. Pure glycerin is not prone to oxidation by the atmosphere under ordinary storage conditions, but decomposes on heating, with the evolution of toxic acrolein. Mixtures of glycerin with water, ethanol, and propylene glycol are chemically stable. Glycerin may crystallize if stored at low temperatures; the crystals do not melt until raised to 20°C. Glycerin should be stored in an airtight container, in a cool, dry, place.

Incompatibilities

Glycerin may explode if mixed with strong oxidizing agents such as chromium trioxide, potassium chlorate, or potassium permanganate. In dilute solution, the reaction proceeds at a slower rate with several oxidation products being formed. Black discoloration of glycerin occurs in the presence of light, on contact with zinc oxide or basic bismuth nitrate.

Bentonite

Synonyms

Mineral soap; Soap clay; Taylorite; Veegum HS; Wilkinite

Molecular Formula

$Al_2O_3.4SiO_2.H_2O$ (359.16)

Characteristics

Bentonite is a crystalline, clay-like mineral, and is available as an odorless, pale buff, or cream to grayish-colored fine powder, which is free from grit. It consists of particles about 50-150 μm in size along with numerous particles about 1-2 μm. Microscopic examination of samples stained with alcoholic methylene blue solution reveals strongly stained blue particles. Bentonite may have a slight earthy taste. Bentonite is a native colloidal hydrated aluminum silicate consisting mainly of montmorillonite, $Al_2O_3.4SiO_2.H_2O$; it may also contain calcium, magnesium, and iron. The average chemical analysis is expressed as oxides and is shown below, in comparison with magnesium aluminum silicate.

Pharmaceutical Applications

Bentonite is a naturally occurring hydrated aluminum silicate used primarily in the formulation of suspensions, gels, and sols, for topical pharmaceutical application. It is also used to suspend powders in aqueous preparations and to prepare cream bases containing oil-in-water emulsifying agents.

Bentonite may also be used in oral pharmaceutical preparations, cosmetics, and food products. In oral preparations, bentonite, and other similar silicate clays, can be used to adsorb cationic drugs and so retard their release. Adsorbents are also used to mask the taste of certain drugs. Bentonite has been investigated as a diagnostic agent for magnetic resonance imaging.

Stability and Storage Conditions

Bentonite is hygroscopic, and sorption of atmospheric water should be avoided. Aqueous bentonite suspensions may be sterilized by autoclaving. The solid material may be sterilized by maintaining it at 170°C for 1 hour after drying at 100°C. Bentonite should be stored in an airtight container in a cool, dry, place.

Incompatibilities

Aqueous bentonite suspensions retain their viscosity above pH 6, but are precipitated by acids. Acid-washed bentonite does not have suspending properties. The addition of alkaline materials, such as magnesium oxide, increases gel formation.

Titanium Dioxide

Synonyms

Anatase titanium dioxide; brookite titanium dioxide; rutile titanium dioxide; titanic anhydride; Tioxide; TiPure.

Molecular Formula

TiO_2 (79.88)

Characteristics

It is white, amorphous, odorless, and tasteless nonhygroscopic powder. Although the average particle size of titanium dioxide powder is less than 1 µm, commercial titanium dioxide generally occurs as aggregated particles of approximately 100-µm diameters. Titanium dioxide may occur in several different crystalline forms: rutile; anatase; and brookite. Of these, rutile and anatase are the only forms of commercial importance. Rutile is the more thermodynamically stable and predominates.

Pharmaceutical Applications

Titanium dioxide is widely used in confectionery, cosmetics, foods, and topical and oral pharmaceutical formulations as a white pigment. Due to its high refractive index titanium dioxide has unique light-scattering properties, which may be exploited in its use as a white pigment and opacifier. In pharmaceutical formulations titanium dioxide is used as a white pigment in film-coating suspensions, sugarcoated tablets, and gelatin capsules. In addition to titanium dioxide being used as a white pigment it may also be admixed with other pigments. Titanium dioxide is also used in dermatological preparations and cosmetics, such as sunscreens.

Stability and Storage Conditions

Titanium dioxide is extremely stable at high temperatures. The exceptional stability is due to the strong bond between the tetravalent titanium ion and the bivalent oxygen ions. Titanium dioxide can however lose small, unweighable amounts of oxygen by interaction with radiant energy. This oxygen can easily recombine again as a part of a reversible photochemical reaction, particularly if there is no oxidizable material available. These small oxygen losses are important because they can cause significant changes in the optical and electrical properties of the pigment. Titanium dioxide should be stored in a well-closed container, protected from light, in a cool, dry, place.

Incompatibilities

Due to a catalytic effect, titanium dioxide may interact with certain active substances.

Isopropyl Myristate

Synonyms

Bisomel; Crodamol IPM; Deltyl Extra; Emcol-IM; Emerest 2314; Estergel; Estol 1514; Isomyst; isopropyl ester of myristic acid; myristic acid isopropyl ester; Plymouth IPM; Promyr; Protachem IPM; Sinnoester MIP; Starfol IPM; Stepan D-50; Tegester; Tetradecanoic acid, 1-methylethyl ester; Unimate IPM; Wickenol 101.

Molecular Formula

$C_{17}H_{34}O_2$ (270.51)

Characteristics

Isopropyl myristate is a clear, colorless, practically odorless liquid of low viscosity, which congeals at about 3°C. It consists of esters of propan-2-ol and saturated high molecular weight fatty acids, principally myristic acid.

Typical Properties

Boiling point : 140.2°C at 266 Pa (2 mmHg)

Flash point : 153.5°C (closed cup)

Solubility : soluble in acetone, chloroform, ethanol, ethyl acetate, fats, fatty alcohols, fixed oils, liquid hydrocarbons, toluene, and waxes. Dissolves many waxes, cholesterol, or lanolin. It is practically insoluble in glycerin, glycols and water.

Pharmaceutical Applications

Isopropyl myristate is a nongreasy emollient that is absorbed readily by the skin. It is used as a component of semisolid bases and as a solvent for many substances applied topically. Applications in topical pharmaceutical and cosmetic formulations include: bath oils; make-up; hair and nail care products; creams; lotions; lip products; shaving products; skin lubricants; deodorants; otic suspensions; and vaginal creams. For example, isopropyl myristate is a self-emulsifying component of a proposed cold cream formula, which is suitable for use as a vehicle for drugs or dermatological actives.

Isopropyl myristate is used as a penetration enhancer for transdermal formulations and has been used in conjunction with therapeutic ultrasound and iontophoresis. It has been used in a water-oil-gel prolonged-release emulsion in which isopropyl myristate is the major ingredient of the oil phase.

Stability and Storage Conditions

Isopropyl myristate is resistant to oxidation and hydrolysis and does not become rancid. It should be stored in a well-closed container in a cool, dry, place and protected from light.

Incompatibilities

When isopropyl myristate comes into contact with rubber, there is a drop in viscosity with concomitant swelling and partial dissolution of the rubber; contact with plastics, e.g., nylon and polyethylene, results in swelling. Isopropyl myristate is incompatible with hard paraffin, producing a granular mixture. It is also incompatible with strong oxidizing agents.

Cetyl alcohol

Synonyms

Crodacol C70; Crodacol C90; Crodacol C95; ethal; ethol; 1-hexadecanol; n-hexadecyl alcohol; palmityl alcohol.

Molecular Formula

$C_{16}H_{34}O$ (242.44)

Characteristics

Cetyl alcohol occurs as waxy, white flakes, granules, cubes, or castings. It has a faint characteristic odor and bland taste. Cetyl alcohol, used in pharmaceutical preparations, is a mixture of solid aliphatic alcohols comprising mainly 1-hexadecanol ($C_{16}H_{34}O$). The USP specifies not less than 90.0% of cetyl alcohol and the remainder consisting chiefly of related alcohols. Commercially, many grades of cetyl alcohol are available as mixtures of cetyl alcohol (60-70%) and stearyl alcohol (20-30%), the remainder being related alcohols.

Pharmaceutical Applications

Cetyl alcohol is widely used in pharmaceuticals and cosmetics, such as, suppositories, modified-release solid dosage forms, emulsions, lotions, creams, and ointments. In suppositories, cetyl alcohol is used to raise the melting point of the base, and in modified-release dosage forms, it may be used to form a permeable barrier coating. In lotions, creams, and ointments, cetyl alcohol is used because of its emollient, water absorptive, and emulsifying properties. It enhances stability, improves texture, and increases consistency. The emollient properties are due to absorption and retention of cetyl alcohol in the epidermis, where it lubricates and softens the skin while imparting a characteristic 'velvety' texture.

Stability and Storage Conditions

Cetyl alcohol is stable in the presence of acids, alkalis, light, and air; it does not become rancid. It should be stored in a well-closed container in a cool, dry, place.

Incompatibilities

Incompatible with strong oxidizing agents

Sorbitan Monooleate

Structural Formula

$$CH_2-R_3$$
$$HC-R_2$$

$R_1 = R_2 = OH$, $R_3 = R$ for sorbitan monoesters,

$R_1 = OH$, $R_2 = R_3 = R$ for sorbitan diesters,

$R_1 = R_2 = R_3 = R$ for sorbitan triesters,

Where $R = (C_{17}H_{35})COO$ for isostearate,

$(C_{11}H_{23})COO$ for laurate,

$(C_{17}H_{33})COO$ for oleate,

$(C_{15}H_{31})COO$ for palmitate,

$(C_{17}H_{35})COO$ for stearate.

The sesqui-esters are equimolar mixtures of monoesters and diesters.

Characteristics

Sorbitan esters occur as cream to amber-colored liquids or solids with a distinctive odor and taste.

Pharmaceutical Applications

Sorbitan monoesters are a series of mixtures of partial esters of sorbitol and its mono- and di-anhydrides with fatty acids. Sorbitan esters are widely used in cosmetics, food products, and pharmaceutical formulations as lipophilic nonionic surfactants. They are mainly used in pharmaceutical formulations as emulsifying agents in the preparation of creams, emulsions, and ointments for topical application. When used alone, sorbitan esters produce stable water-in-oil emulsions and microemulsions but are frequently used in combination with varying proportions of a polysorbate to produce water-in-oil or oil-in- water emulsions or creams of varying consistencies.

Sorbitan monolaurate, sorbitan monopalmitate and sorbitan trioleate have also been used at a concentration of 0.01-0.05% w/v in the preparation of an emulsion for intramuscular administration.

Stability and Storage Conditions

Gradual soap formation occurs with strong acids or bases; sorbitan esters are stable in weak acids or bases. Sorbitan esters should be stored in a well-closed container in a cool, dry, place.

Safety

Sorbitan esters are widely used in cosmetics, food products, and oral and topical pharmaceutical formulations and are generally regarded as nontoxic and nonirritant materials. However, there have been occasional reports of hypersensitive skin reactions following the topical application of products containing sorbitan esters. When heated to decomposition the sorbitan esters emit acrid smoke and irritating fumes.

The WHO has set an estimated acceptable daily intake of sorbitan monopalmitate, monostearate and tristearate, and sorbitan monolaurate, and monooleate at up to 25 mg/kg body-weight calculated as total sorbitan esters.

Polyoxyethylene stearates

Synonyms

Ethoxylated fatty acid esters; macrogol stearates; Marlosol; PEG fatty acid esters; PEG stearates; polyethylene glycol stearates; polyoxyethylene glycol stearates.

Characteristics

Polyoxyethylene stearates are nonionic surfactants produced by polyethoxylation of stearic acid. Two systems of nomenclature are used for these materials. The number '8' in the names 'poloxyl 8 stearate' or 'polyoxyethylene 8 stearate' refers to the approximate polymer length in oxyethylene units. The same material may also be designated 'polyoxyethylene glycol 400 stearate' or 'macrogol stearate 400' in which case, the number '400' refers to the average molecular weight of the polymer chain.

Pharmaceutical Applications

Polyoxyethylene stearates are generally used as emulsifiers in oil-in-water-type creams and lotions. Their hydrophilicity or lipophilicity depends on the number of ethylene oxide units present: the larger the number, the greater the hydrophilic properties. Polyoxyl 40 stearate has also been used as an emulsifying agent in intravenous infusions. Polyoxyethylene stearates are particularly useful as emulsifying agents when astringent salts or other strong electrolytes are present. They can also be blended with other surfactants to obtain any hydrophilic-lipophilic balance for lotions or ointment formulations.

Stearic Acid

Nonproprietary Names : BP: Stearic acid, JP: Stearic acid, USP: Stearic acid

Synonyms

Acidum stearicum; Crodacid; Crosterene; Glycon S-90; Hystrene; Industrene; Kortacid 1895; Pristerene.

Molecular Formula

$C_{18}H_{36}O_2$ (284.47)

Characteristics

Stearic acid is a hard, white or faintly yellow colored, somewhat glossy, crystalline solid or a white, or yellowish white, powder. It has a slight odor and taste suggesting tallow.

Pharmaceutical Applications

Stearic acid is widely used in oral and topical pharmaceutical formulations. It is mainly used in oral formulations as a tablet and capsule lubricant although it may also be used as a binder, or in combination with shellac as a tablet coating.

In topical formulations, stearic acid is used as an emulsifying and solubilizing agent. When partially neutralized with alkalis or triethanolamine, stearic acid is used in the preparation of creams. The partially neutralized stearic acid forms a creamy base when mixed with 5-15 times its own weight of aqueous liquid, the appearance and plasticity of the cream being determined by the proportion of alkali used. It is used as the hardening agent in glycerin suppositories.

Stearic acid is also widely used in cosmetics and food products.

Stability and Storage Conditions

Stearic acid is a stable material; an antioxidant may also be added to it. The bulk material should be stored in a well-closed container in a cool, dry, place.

Incompatibilities

Stearic acid is incompatible with most metal hydroxides and may be incompatible with oxidizing agents. Insoluble stearates are formed with many metals; ointment bases made with stearic acid may show evidence of drying out or lumpiness due to such a reaction when compounded with zinc or calcium salts.

A number of differential scanning calorimetry studies have investigated the compatibility of stearic acid with drugs. Although such laboratory studies have suggested incompatibilities, e.g., naproxen, they may not necessarily be applicable to formulated products. Stearic acid has been reported to cause pitting in the film- coating of tablets coated using an aqueous film-coating technique; the pitting was found to be a function of the melting point of the stearic acid.

Isopropyl palmitate

Nonproprietary Names : BP: Isopropyl palmitate, PhEur: Isopropylis palmitas, USP: Isopropyl palmitate

Synonyms

Crodamol IPP; Deltyl; Deltyl Prime; Emcol-IP; hexadecanoic acid isopropyl ester; hexadecanoic acid 1-methylethyl ester; Isopal; Isopalm; isopropyl hexadecanoate; Kessco IPP; palmitic acid isopropyl ester; Plymouth IPP; Propal; Protachem IPP; Stepan D-70; Tegester Isopalm; Unimate IPP.

Molecular Formula

$C_{19}H_{38}O_2$ (298.51)

Characteristics

Isopropyl palmitate is a clear, colorless to pale yellow-colored, practically odorless viscous liquid, which solidifies at less than 16°C.

Typical Properties

Boiling point : 160°C at 266 Pa (2 mmHg)

Freezing point : 13-15°C

Solubility : soluble in acetone, chloroform, ethanol, ethyl acetate, mineral oil, propan-2-ol, silicone oils, vegetable oils, and aliphatic and aromatic hydrocarbons; practically insoluble in glycerin, glycols, and water.

Pharmaceutical Applications

Isopropyl palmitate is a nonoleaginous emollient with good spreading characteristics used in topical pharmaceutical formulations and cosmetics such as: bath oils; creams; lotions; make-up; hair care products; deodorants; lip products; suntan preparations; and pressed powders. Isopropyl palmitate has also been used in a controlled-release percutaneous film.

Stability and Storage Conditions

Isopropyl palmitate is resistant to oxidation and hydrolysis and does not become rancid. It should be stored in a well-closed container, above 16°C, and protected from light.

Propylene Glycol

Nonproprietary Names : BP: Propylene glycol, JP: Propylene glycol, PhEur: Propylenglycolum, USP: Propylene glycol

Synonyms

1,2-Dihydroxypropane; 2-hydroxypropanol; methyl ethylene glycol; methyl glycol; propane-1,2-diol.

Molecular Formula

$C_3H_8O_2$ (76.1)

Pharmaceutical Applications

Propylene glycol has become widely used as a solvent, extractant, and preservative in a variety of parenteral and nonparenteral pharmaceutical formulations. It is a better general solvent than glycerin and dissolves a wide variety of materials, such as corticosteroids, phenols, sulfa drugs, barbiturates, vitamins (A and D), most alkaloids, and many local anesthetics.

As an antiseptic it is similar to ethanol, and against molds it is similar to glycerin and only slightly less effective than ethanol. Propylene glycol is commonly used as a plasticizer in aqueous film-coating formulations. Propylene glycol is also used in cosmetics and in the food industry as a carrier for emulsifiers and as a vehicle for flavors in preference to ethanol, since its lack of volatility provides a more uniform flavor.

Stability and Storage Conditions

At cool temperatures, propylene glycol is stable in a well- closed container, but at high temperatures, in the open, it tends to oxidize, giving rise to products such as propionaldehyde, lactic acid, pyruvic acid, and acetic acid. Propylene glycol is chemically stable when mixed with ethanol (95%), glycerin, or water; aqueous solutions may be sterilized by autoclaving.

Propylene glycol is hygroscopic and should be stored in a well- closed container, protected from light, in a cool, dry, place.

Incompatibilities

Propylene glycol is incompatible with oxidizing reagents such as potassium permanganate.

White beeswax

Nonproprietary Names : BP: White beeswax, JP: White beeswax, PhEur: Cera alba, USP: White wax

Synonyms

901 (Beeswax); bleached wax.

Molecular Formula

White wax is the chemically bleached form of natural beeswax. Beeswax consists of 70-75% of a mixture of various esters of straight-chain monohydric alcohols with even-number carbon chains from C_{24}-C_{36} esterified with straight-chain acids, which also have even numbers of carbon atoms up to C_{36} together with some C_{18} hydroxy acids. The chief ester is myricyl palmitate. Also present are free acids (about 14%) and carbohydrates (about 12%) as well as approximately 1% free wax alcohols and stearic esters of fatty acids.

Characteristics

White wax consists of tasteless, white or slightly yellow-colored sheets or fine granules with some translucence. Odor is similar to yellow wax although it is less intense.

Pharmaceutical Applications

White wax is a chemically bleached form of yellow wax and is used in similar applications, such as to increase the consistency of creams and ointments, and to stabilize water-in-oil emulsions. White wax is also used to polish sugarcoated tablets and to adjust the melting point of suppositories.

White wax is also used in controlled-release systems. White beeswax microspheres may be used in oral-dosage forms to retard the absorption of an active ingredient from the stomach, allowing the majority of absorption to occur in the intestinal tract. Wax coatings can also be used to affect the release of drug from ion-exchange resin beads.

Stability and Storage Conditions

When heated above 150°C esterification occurs with a consequent lowering of acid value and elevation of melting point. White wax is stable when stored in a well-closed container, protected from light.

Incompatibilities : Incompatible with oxidizing agents.

Paraffin wax

Nonproprietary Names : BP: Hard paraffin, JP: Paraffin, PhEur: Paraffin solidum, USP: Paraffin

Synonyms

Hard wax; paraffinum durum; paraffinum solidum; paraffin wax.

Molecular Formula

Paraffin is a purified mixture of solid saturated hydrocarbons having the general formula C_nH_{2n+2}, and is obtained from petroleum or shale oil.

Characteristics

Paraffin is an odorless and tasteless, translucent, colorless, or white solid. It feels slightly greasy to the touch and may show a brittle fracture. Microscopically, it is a mixture of bundles of microcrystals. Paraffin burns with a luminous, sooty flame. When melted, paraffin is essentially free from fluorescence in daylight; a slight odor may be apparent.

Typical Properties

Density : 0.84-0.89 g/cm^3 at 20°C

Melting point : various grades with different specified melting ranges are commercially available.

Solubility : soluble in chloroform, ether, volatile oils, and most warm fixed oils; slightly soluble in ethanol; practically insoluble in acetone, ethanol (95%), and water. Paraffin can be mixed with most waxes if melted and cooled.

Pharmaceutical Applications

Paraffin is mainly used in topical pharmaceutical formulations as a component of creams and ointments. In ointments, it may be used to increase the melting point of a formulation or to add stiffness. Paraffin is additionally used as a coating agent for capsules and tablets and is used in some food applications. Paraffin coatings can also be used to affect the release of drug from ion-exchange resin beads.

Stability and Storage Conditions

Paraffin is stable, although repeated melting and congealing may alter its physical properties. Paraffin should be stored at a temperature not exceeding 40°C in well-closed container.

Mineral oil

Nonproprietary Names : BP: Liquid paraffin, JP: Liquid paraffin, PhEur: Paraffinum liquidum, USP: Mineral oil

Synonyms

Alboline; Drakeol; Glymol; heavy mineral oil; liquid petrolatum; Nujol; paraffin oil; white mineral oil.

Molecular Formula

Mineral oil is a mixture of refined liquid saturated aliphatic (C_{14} to C_{18}) and cyclic hydrocarbons obtained from petroleum.

Characteristics

Mineral oil is a transparent, colorless, viscous oily liquid, free from fluorescence in daylight. It is practically tasteless and odorless when cold, and has a faint odor of petroleum when heated.

Typical Properties

Boiling point : > 360°C

Flash point : 210-224°C

Pour point : -12.2 to -9.4°C

Refractive index : n_D^{20} = 1.4756-1.4800

Solubility : practically insoluble in ethanol (95%), glycerin, and water; soluble in acetone, benzene, chloroform, carbon disulfide, ether, and petroleum ether. It is miscible with volatile and fixed oils, with the exception of castor oil.

Pharmaceutical Applications

Mineral oil is used primarily as an excipient in topical pharmaceutical formulations where its emollient properties are exploited as an ingredient in ointment bases. It is additionally used in oil-in-water emulsions, as a solvent, and as a lubricant in capsule and tablet formulations, and to a limited extent, as a mold-release agent for cocoa butter suppositories. More recently it has been used in the preparation of microspheres. Therapeutically, mineral oil has been used as a laxative. It is indigestible and thus has limited absorption. Mineral oil is used in ophthalmic formulations for its lubricant properties. It is also used in cosmetics and food products.

Stability and Storage Conditions

Mineral oil undergoes oxidation when exposed to heat and light. Oxidation begins with the formation of peroxides, exhibiting 'induction period'. Under ordinary conditions, the induction period may take months or years. However, once a trace of peroxide is formed, further oxidation is autocatalytic and proceeds very rapidly. Oxidation results in the formation of aldehydes and organic acids, which impart taste and odor. Stabilizers may be added to retard oxidation; butylated hydroxyanisole, butylated hydroxytoluene, and tocopherol being the most commonly used antioxidants. Mineral oil may be sterilized by dry heat.

Mineral oil should be stored in an airtight container, protected from light, in a cool, dry, place.

Incompatibilities

It is incompatible with strong oxidizing agents.

Cetyl Esters Wax

Nonprop rietary Names USP : Cetyl esters wax

Synonyms

Cera cetyla; Crodamol SS; Liponate SPS; Protachem MST; Ritaceti; Ritachol SS; spermaceti wax replacement; Starfol Wax CG; synthetic spermaceti.

Molecular Formula

$C_nH_{2n}O_2$ (470-490)

Where n = 26-38.

Cetyl esters wax as a mixture consisting primarily of esters of saturated fatty alcohols (C_{14}-C_{18}) and saturated fatty acids (C_{14}-C_{18}).

Characteristics

Cetyl esters wax occurs as white to off-white, somewhat translucent flakes (typically in the range of 5 μm to several millimeters in the largest dimension), having a crystalline structure and a pearly luster when caked. It has a faint, aromatic odor and a bland, mild taste.

Pharmaceutical Applications

Cetyl esters wax is a stiffening agent and emollient used in creams and ointments as a replacement for naturally occurring spermaceti.

Cetyl esters wax is hydrophobic, and has been proposed as a suitable component of an ophthalmic gelatin based, controlled-release delivery matrix. The physical properties of cetyl esters wax vary greatly from manufacturer to manufacturer due to differences between the mixtures of fatty acids and fatty alcohol esters that are used. Differences between products appear most obviously in the melting point, which can range from 43-47°C (USP range) to 51-55°C, depending on the mixture. Materials with a high melting point tend to contain predominantly cetyl and stearyl palmitates.

Stability and Storage Conditions

Store in a well-closed container in a cool, dry, place. Avoid exposure to excessive heat (over 40°C).

Incompatibilities

It is incompatible with strong acids or bases.

White Wax

Nonproprietary Names BP : White beeswax, JP: White beeswax, USP: White wax

Synonyms

Bleached wax

Molecular Formula

White wax is the chemically bleached form of natural beeswax, Beeswax consists of 70-75% of a mixture of various esters of straight-chain monohydric alcohols with even-number carbon chains from C_{24}-C_{36} esterified with straight-chain acids which also have even numbers of carbon atoms up to C_{36} together with some C_{18} hydroxy acids. The chief ester is myricyl palmitate. Also present are free acids (about 14%) and carbohydrates (about 12%) as well as approximately 1% free wax alcohols and stearic esters of fatty acids.

Characteristics

White wax consists of tasteless, white or slightly yellow-colored sheets or fine granules with some translucence. Odor is similar to yellow wax although it is less intense.

Solubility : soluble in chloroform, ether, fixed oils, volatile oils, and warm carbon disulfide; sparingly soluble in ethanol (95%); practically insoluble in water.

Pharmaceutical Applications

White wax is a chemically bleached form of yellow wax and is used in similar applications, such as to increase the consistency of creams and ointments, and to stabilize water-in-oil emulsions. White wax is also used to polish sugarcoated tablets and to adjust the melting point of suppositories.

White wax is also used in controlled-release systems. White beeswax microspheres may be used in oral-dosage forms to retard the absorption of an active ingredient from the stomach, allowing the majority of absorption to occur in the intestinal tract. Wax coatings can also be used to affect the release of drug from ion-exchange resin beads.

Stability and Storage Conditions

When heated above 150°C esterification occurs with a consequent lowering of acid value and elevation of melting point. White wax is stable when stored in a well-closed container, protected from light.

Incompatibilities

Incompatible with oxidizing agents

Cholesterol

Nonproprietary Names BP : Cholesterol, JP: Cholesterol, PhEur: Cholesterolum, USP: Cholesterol

Synonyms

Cholesterin.

Molecular Formula

$C_{27}H_{46}O$ (386.67)

Characteristics

It is white or faintly yellow, almost odorless, needles, powder, or granules. On prolonged exposure to light and air cholesterol acquires a yellow to tan color.

Pharmaceutical Applications

Cholesterol is used in cosmetics and topical pharmaceutical formulations at concentrations between 0.3-5.0% w/w as an emulsifying agent. It imparts water-absorbing power to an ointment and has emollient activity. Cholesterol additionally has a physiological role.

Stability and Storage Conditions

Cholesterol is stable and should be stored in a well-closed container, protected from light.

Incompatibilities

Precipitated by digitonin.

Propylparaben

Nonproprietary Names BP : Propyl hydroxybenzoate, JP: Propyl parahydroxybenzoate, PhEur: Propylis parahydroxybenzoas, USP: Propylparaben

Synonyms

Chemocide PK; 4-hydroxybenzoic acid propyl ester; Nipasol M; propagin; Propyl chemosept; propyl p-hydroxybenzoate; Propyl parasept; Solbrol P; Tegosept P.

Molecular Formula

$C_{10}H_{12}O_3$ (180.20)

Characteristics

Propylparaben exhibits antimicrobial activity between pH 4-8. Preservative efficacy decreases with increasing pH due to the formation of the phenolate anion. Parabens are more active against yeasts and molds than against bacteria. They are also more active against Gram-positive than against Gram-negative bacteria. The activity of the parabens increases with increasing chain length of the alkyl moiety; solubility however decreases. Activity may be improved by using combinations of parabens since additive effects occur. Propylparaben has thus been used with methylparaben in parenteral preparations and is used with combinations of other parabens in topical and oral formulations. Activity has also been reported to be improved by the addition of other excipients.

Pharmaceutical Applications

Propylparaben is widely used as an antimicrobial preservative in cosmetics, food products, and pharmaceutical formulations. It may be used alone, in combination with other paraben esters, or with other antimicrobial agents. In cosmetics it is the second most frequently used preservative. The parabens are effective over a wide pH range and have a broad spectrum of antimicrobial activity although they are most effective against yeasts and molds.

Due to the poor solubility of the parabens, paraben salts, particularly the sodium salt, are frequently used in formulations. This may cause the pH of poorly buffered formulations to become more alkaline.

Propylparaben (0.02%) together with methylparaben (0.18%) has been used for the preservation of various parenteral pharmaceutical formulations.

Stability and Storage Conditions

Aqueous propylparaben solutions at pH 3-6 can be sterilized by autoclaving, without decomposition. At pH 3-6 aqueous solutions are stable (less than 10% decomposition) for up to about 4 years at room temperature while solutions at pH 8 or above are subject to rapid hydrolysis (10% or more after about 60 days at room temperature).

Incompatibilities

The antimicrobial activity of propylparaben is considerably reduced in the presence of nonionic surfactants as a result of micellization. Absorption of propylparaben by plastics has been reported, with the amount-absorbed dependent upon the type of plastic and the vehicle. Magnesium aluminum silicate, magnesium trisilicate, yellow iron oxide, and ultramarine blue have also been reported to absorb propylparaben, thereby reducing preservative efficacy.

Propylparaben is discolored in the presence of iron and is subject to hydrolysis by weak alkalis and strong acids.

Methylparabane

Nonproprietary Names: BP : Methyl hydroxybenzoate, JP: Methyl parahydroxybenzoate, PhEur: Methylis parahydroxybenzoas, USP: Methylparaben

Synonyms

4-hydroxybenzoic acid methyl ester; Methyl Chemosept; methyl p-hydroxybenzoate; Methyl Parasept; Nipagin M; Solbrol M; Tegosept M.

Molecular Formula

$C_8H_8O_3$ (152.15)

Characteristics

Methylparaben exhibits antimicrobial activity between pH 4-8. Preservative efficacy decreases with increasing pH due to the formation of the phenolate anion. Parabens are more active against yeasts and molds than against bacteria. They are also more active against Gram- positive bacteria than against Gram-negative bacteria.

Methylparaben is the least active of the parabens; antimicrobial activity increases with increasing chain length of the alkyl moiety. Activity may be improved by using combinations of parabens, since additive effects occur. Therefore, combinations of methyl, ethyl, propyl, and butylparaben are often used together. Activity has also been reported to be enhanced by the addition of other excipients such as: propylene glycol (2-5%); phenylethyl alcohol; and edetic acid. Activity may also be enhanced, due to synergistic effects, by using combinations of parabens with other antimicrobial preservatives such as imidurea. The hydrolysis product, *p*-hydroxybenzoic acid, has practically no antimicrobial activity.

Pharmaceutical Applications

Methylparaben is widely used as an antimicrobial preservative in cosmetics, food products, and pharmaceutical formulations. It may be used either alone, in combination with other parabens, or with other antimicrobial agents. In cosmetics, methylparaben is the most frequently used antimicrobial preservative. Due to the poor solubility of the parabens, paraben salts, particularly the sodium salt, are frequently used in formulations. However, this raises the pH of poorly buffered formulations.

Methylparaben (0.18%) together with propylparaben (0.02%) has been used for the preservation of various parenteral pharmaceutical formulations.

Stability and Storage Conditions

Aqueous solutions of methylparaben, at pH 3-6, may be sterilized by autoclaving at 120°C for 20 minutes, without decomposition. Aqueous solutions at pH 3-6 are stable (less than 10% decomposition) for up to about 4 years at room temperature, while aqueous solutions at pH 8 or above are subject to rapid hydrolysis (10% or more after about 60 days storage at room temperature).

Methylparaben should be stored in a well-closed container in a cool, dry, place.

Incompatibilities

The antimicrobial activity of methylparaben and other parabens is considerably reduced in the presence of nonionic surfactants, such as polysorbate 80, as a result of micellization.

However, propylene glycol (10%) has been shown to potentiate the antimicrobial activity of the parabens in the presence of nonionic surfactants and prevents the interaction between methylparaben and polysorbate 80.

Incompatibilities with other substances such as bentonite, magnesium trisilicate, talc, tragacanth, sodium alginate, essential oils, sorbitol, and atropine have been reported.

Absorption of methylparaben by plastics has also been reported; the amount absorbed is dependent upon the type of plastic and the vehicle. It has been claimed that low- and high-density polyethylene bottles do not absorb methylparaben.

Methylparaben is discolored in the presence of iron and is subject to hydrolysis by weak alkalis and strong acids.

Glyceryl Monostearate

Nonproprietary Names : BP: Glyceryl monostearate 40-50, JP: Glyceryl monostearate, PhEur: Glyceryli monostearas, USP: Glyceryl monostearate

Synonyms

Abracol SLG; Admul; Advawax 140; Cefatin; Celinhol-A; Citomulgin M; Cyclochem GMS; Dermgine; Diastearate; Drewmulse TP, V, AA; Emerest 2401; Emcol CA, MSK; Emul P.7; Estol 603, 1473; glycerine monostearate; glycerol monostearate; glycerol stearate; glyceryl stearate; GMS; Grocor 5500, 6000; Hodag GMS; Imwitor 191, 900K; Kessco 40; Lipo GMS 410, 450, 600; monostearin; Myvaplex 600P; Ogeen 515, GRB, M, MAV; Orbon; Protachem GMS-450; Sedetine; stearic monoglyceride; Rita- GMS; Simulsol 165; Tegin 503, 515; Unimate GMS; USAF KE-7; Witconol MS, MST.

Molecular Formula

$C_{21}H_{42}O_4$ (358.6)

Characteristics

The USP describes glyceryl monostearate as consisting of not less than 90% of monoglycerides, chiefly glyceryl monostearate ($C_{21}H_{42}O_4$) and glyceryl monopalmitate ($C_{19}H_{38}O_4$). The PhEur describes glyceryl monostearate 40-50 as a mixture of monoacylglycerols, mostly stearoyl- and palmitic acids, together with quantities of di- and tri-acylglycerols. It contains 40-50% of 1-monoacylglycerols, and not more than 6% of free glycerin.

Glyceryl monostearate is a white to cream-colored, wax-like solid in the form of beads, flakes, or powder. It is waxy to the touch and has a slight fatty odor and taste.

Typical Properties

A wide variety of glyceryl monostearate grades are commercially available, including self-emulsifying grades, which contain small amounts of soap or other surfactants. Most grades are tailored for specific applications or made to user specifications and thus have varied physical properties.

Melting point : 55-60°C

Flash point : 240°C

HLB value : 3.8

Solubility : soluble in hot ethanol, ether, chloroform, hot acetone, mineral oil, and fixed oils. Practically insoluble in water, but may be dispersed in water with the aid of a small amount of soap or other surfactant.

Pharmaceutical Applications

Glyceryl monostearate is used as a nonionic emulsifier, stabilizer, emollient, and plasticizer in a variety of food, pharmaceutical, and cosmetic applications. It acts as an effective stabilizer, i.e., as a mutual solvent for polar and nonpolar compounds, which may form water-in-oil or oil-in-water emulsions. These properties also make it useful as a dispersing agent for pigments in oils or solids in fats, or as a solvent for phospholipids, such as lecithin.

Glyceryl monostearate is a lubricant for tablet manufacturing and may be used to form sustained-release matrices for solid dosage forms. Sustained-release applications include the formulation of pellets for tablets or suppositories and the preparation of a veterinary bolus. It has also been used as a matrix ingredient for a biodegradable, implantable, controlled-release dosage form.

Stability and Storage Conditions

Glyceryl monostearate increases in acid value upon aging, if stored at warm temperatures, due to the saponification of the ester with trace amounts of water. Effective antioxidants that may be added are butylated hydroxytoluene and propyl gallate.

Glyceryl monostearate should be stored in a tightly closed container in a cool, dry place, and protected from light.

Incompatibilities

The self-emulsifying grades of glyceryl monostearate are incompatible with acidic substances.

Lanolin

Nonproprietary Names BP : Wool fat, JP: Purified lanolin, PhEur: Adeps lanae, USP: Lanolin

Synonyms

Corona; lanolin anhydrous; purified lanolin; refined wool fat

Molecular Formula

The USP describes lanolin as the purified wax-like substance obtained from the wool of the sheep, *Ovis aries* Linné (Fam. Bovidae), that has been cleaned, decolorized, and deodorized. It contains not more than 0.25% w/w of water and may contain 0.02% w/w of a suitable antioxidant; the PhEur specifies up to 200 ppm of butylated hydroxytoluene as an antioxidant.

Characteristics

Lanolin is a pale yellow colored, unctuous, waxy substance with a faint, characteristic odor. Melted lanolin is a clear or almost clear, yellow liquid.

Solubility : freely soluble in benzene, chloroform, ether, and petroleum spirit; sparingly soluble in cold ethanol (95%), more soluble in boiling ethanol (95%); practically insoluble in water.

Pharmaceutical Applications

Lanolin is widely used in topical pharmaceutical formulations and cosmetics.

Lanolin may be used as a hydrophobic vehicle and in the preparation of water-in-oil creams and ointments. When mixed with suitable vegetable oils or with soft paraffin it produces emollient creams, which penetrate the skin and hence facilitate the absorption of drugs. Lanolin mixes with about twice its own weight of water, without separation, to produce stable emulsions, which do not readily become rancid on storage.

Stability and Storage Conditions

Lanolin may gradually undergo autoxidation during storage. To inhibit this process the inclusion of butylated hydroxytoluene is permitted as an antioxidant. Exposure to excessive or prolonged heating may cause anhydrous lanolin to darken in color and develop a strong rancid-like odor. However, lanolin may be sterilized by dry heat at 150°C. Sterile ophthalmic ointments containing lanolin may be sterilized by filtration or by exposure to gamma irradiation.

Lanolin should be stored in a well-filled, well-closed container protected from light, in a cool, dry, place. Normal storage life is 2 years.

Incompatibilities

Lanolin may contain pro-oxidants, which may affect the stability of certain active drugs.

Lactic Acid

Nonproprietary Names BP : Lactic acid, JP: Lactic acid, PhEur: Acidum lacticum, USP: Lactic acid

Synonyms

Eco-Lac; 2-hydroxypropanoic acid; 2-hydroxypropionic acid; DL-lactic acid; milk acid; Patlac LA; Purac 88 PH; racemic lactic acid.

Molecular Formula

$C_3H_6O_3$ (90.08)

Pharmaceutical Applications

Lactic acid is used in beverages, foods, cosmetics, and pharmaceuticals as an acidifying agent and acidulant.

In topical formulations, particularly cosmetics, it is used for its softening and conditioning effect on the skin. Lactic acid may also be used in the production of biodegradable polymers and microspheres, such as poly (D-lactic acid), used in drug delivery systems.

Lactic acid is also used as a food preservative and in injections, in the form of lactate, as a source of bicarbonate for the treatment of metabolic acidosis; as a spermicidal agent; in pessaries for the treatment of leucorrhoea; in infant feeds; and in topical formulations for the treatment of warts.

Stability and Storage Conditions

Lactic acid is hygroscopic and will form condensation products, such as polylactic acids on contact with water; the equilibrium between the polylactic acids and lactic acid is dependent on concentration and temperature. At elevated temperatures lactic acid will form lactide, which is readily hydrolyzed back to lactic acid.

Lactic acid should be stored in a well-closed container in a cool and dry place.

Incompatibilities

It is incompatible with oxidizing agents, iodides, and albumin. Reacts violently with hydrofluoric acid and nitric acid.

Triethanolamine

Nonproprietary Names BP : Triethanolamine, USP: Trolamine

Synonyms

Daltogen; Sterolamide; Thiofaco T-35; TEA; triethylolamine; trihydro-xytriethylamine; tris(hydroxyethyl)amine.

Molecular Formula

$C_6H_{15}NO_3$ (149.19)

Characteristics

Triethanolamine is a clear, colorless to pale yellow-colored viscous liquid having a slight ammoniacal odor.

Pharmaceutical Applications

Triethanolamine is widely used in topical pharmaceutical formulations primarily in the formation of emulsions. When mixed in equimolar proportions with a fatty acid, such as stearic acid or oleic acid, triethanolamine forms an anionic soap which may be used as an emulsifying agent to produce fine-grained, stable oil-in-water emulsions with a pH of about 8. Concentrations that are typically used for emulsification are 2-4% of triethanolamine and 2-5 times that of fatty acids. In the case of mineral oils, 5% of triethanolamine will be needed with an appropriate increase in the amount of fatty acid used. Preparations, which contain triethanolamine soaps, tend to darken on storage. However, avoiding exposure to light and contact with metals and metal ions may reduce discoloration.

Triethanolamine is also used in salt formation for injectable solutions and in topical analgesic preparations. Other general uses are as buffers, solvents, polymer plasticizers, and humectants.

Stability and Storage Conditions

Triethanolamine may turn brown on exposure to air and light. The 85% grade of triethanolamine tends to stratify below 15°C; warming and mixing before use can restore homegeneity. Triethanolamine should be stored in an airtight container protected from light, in a cool and dry place.

Incompatibilities

Triethanolamine is a tertiary amine, which contains hydroxyl groups. It is thus capable of undergoing reactions typical of tertiary amines and alcohols. Triethanolamine will react with mineral acids to form crystalline salts and esters. With the higher fatty acids, triethanolamine forms salts, which are soluble in water and have characteristics of soaps. Triethanolamine will also react with copper to form complex salts. Discoloration and precipitation can take place in the presence of heavy metal salts.

Triethanolamine can react with reagents such as thionyl chloride to replace the hydroxy groups with halogens. The products of these reactions are very toxic, resembling other nitrogen mustards.

Vegetable Oil

Nonproprietary Names BP : Hydrogenated vegetable oil, JP: Hydrogenated oil, USP: Hydrogenated vegetable oil, type I

Synonyms

Hard fat, Hydrogenated cottonseed oil: Lubritab; Sterotex, Hydrogenated palm oil, Hydrogenated soybean oil: Sterotex HM.

Structural Formula

$R_1COOCH_2\_CH(OOCR_2)-CH_2OOCR_3$

Where R_1, R_2, and R_3 are mainly C_{15} and C_{17}.

Characteristics

Hydrogenated vegetable oil is a mixture of triglycerides of fatty acids. Two types, which are defined in the USP, are characterized by their physical properties.

Hydrogenated vegetable oil, type I occurs in various forms, e.g., fine powder, flakes, or pellets. The color of the material depends on the manufacturing process and the form. In general, the material is white to yellowish-white with the powder grades appearing white-colored than the coarser grades.

Typical Properties

Density (tapped) : 0.57 g/cm^3

Melting point : 61-66°C

Particle size distribution : 85% < 177 μm, 25% < 74 μm in size. Average particle size is 104 μm.

Solubility : soluble in chloroform, petroleum spirit, and hot propan-2-ol; practically insoluble in water.

Pharmaceutical Applications

Hydrogenated vegetable oil, type I is used as a lubricant in tablet and capsule formulations. It is used at concentrations of 1-6% w/w, usually in combination with talc. It may also be used as an auxiliary binder in tablet formulations.

Hydrogenated vegetable oil, type I is additionally used as the matrix-forming material in lipophilic-based controlled-release formulations; it may also be used as a coating aid in controlled-release formulations.

Other uses of hydrogenated vegetable oil, type I include: as a viscosity modifier in the preparation of oil-based liquid and semisolid formulations; in the preparation of suppositories, to reduce the sedimentation of suspended components and to improve the solidification process; and in the formulation of liquid and semisolid fills for hard-gelatin capsules.

Fully hydrogenated vegetable oil products may also be used as alternatives to hard waxes in cosmetics and topical pharmaceutical formulations.

Stability and Storage Conditions

Hydrogenated vegetable oil, type I is a stable material; typically it is assigned a 2-year shelf life. The bulk material should be stored in a well-closed container in a cool, dry, place.

Incompatibilities

Incompatible with strong oxidizing agents

Castor Oil

Nonproprietary Names USP : Hydrogenated castor oil

Synonyms

Castorwax; Castorwax MP 70; Castorwax MP 80; Opalwax; Simulsol.

Molecular Formula

$C_{57}O_9H_{110}$ (939.50)

The USP describes hydrogenated castor oil as the refined, bleached, hydrogenated, and deodorized castor oil, consisting mainly of the triglyceride of hydroxystearic acid.

Pharmaceutical Applications

Hydrogenated castor oil is a hard, high melting point wax used in oral and topical pharmaceutical formulations.

In topical formulations, hydrogenated castor oil is used to provide stiffness to creams and emulsions.

In oral formulations, hydrogenated castor oil is used to prepare sustained release tablet and capsule preparations; the hydrogenated castor oil may be used as a coat or to form a solid matrix. Hydrogenated castor oil is additionally used to lubricate the die walls of tablet presses; it is similarly used as a lubricant in food processing.

Hydrogenated castor oil is also used in cosmetics.

Stability and Storage Conditions

Hydrogenated castor oil is stable at temperatures up to 150°C.

Clear, stable, chloroform solutions containing up to 15% w/v of hydrogenated castor oil may be produced. Hydrogenated castor oil may also be dissolved at temperatures greater than 90°C in polar solvents and mixtures of aromatic and polar solvents but the hydrogenated castor oil precipitates out on cooling below 90°C.

Store in a well-closed container in a cool and dry place.

Incompatibilities

Hydrogenated castor oil is compatible with most natural vegetable and animal waxes.

Ethylenediaminetetraacetic Acid

Nonproprietary Names BP : Edetic acid, USP: Edetic acid

Synonyms

Edathamil; EDTA; ethylenediaminetetraacetic acid; Questric acid 5286; Sequestrene AA; tetracemic acid; Versene Acid.

Molecular Formula

$C_{10}H_{16}N_2O_8$ (292.24)

Characteristics

Edetic acid occurs as a white crystalline powder.

Pharmaceutical Applications

Edetic acid and edetate salts are used in pharmaceutical formulations, cosmetics, and foods as chelating agents; that is, they form stable water-soluble complexes (chelates) with alkaline earth and heavy metal ions. The chelated form has few of the properties of the free ion, and for this reason-chelating agents are often described as 'removing' ions from solution; this process is also called sequestering. The stability of the metal-edetate complex depends on the metal ion involved and also on the pH. The calcium chelate is relatively weak and will preferentially chelate heavy metals, such as iron, copper, and lead, with the release of calcium ions.

Edetic acid and edetates possess some antimicrobial activity but are most frequently used in combination with other antimicrobial preservatives due to their synergistic effects. Many solutions used for the cleaning, storage, and wetting of contact lenses thus contain disodium edetate. Typically, edetic acid and edetates are used in concentrations of 0.01-0.1% w/v as antimicrobial preservative synergists.

Stability and Storage Conditions

Although edetic acid is fairly stable in the solid state, edetate salts are more stable than the free acid, which decarboxylates if heated above 150°C. Disodium edetate dihydrate loses water of crystallization when heated to 120°C. Edetate calcium disodium is slightly hygroscopic and should be protected from moisture.

Aqueous solutions of edetic acid or edetate salts may be sterilized by autoclaving, and should be stored in an alkali-free container.

Edetic acid and edetates should be stored in well-closed containers in a cool, dry, place.

Incompatibilities

Edetic acid and edetates are incompatible with strong oxidizing agents, strong bases, and polyvalent metal ions such as copper, nickel, and copper alloy.

Edetic acid and disodium edetate behave as weak acids, displacing carbon dioxide from carbonates and reacting with metals to form hydrogen.

Other incompatibilities include the inactivation of certain types of insulin due to the chelation of zinc, and the chelation of trace metals in TPN solutions following the addition of TPN additives stabilized with disodium edetate. Calcium disodium edetate has also been reported to be incompatible with amphotericin and with hydralazine hydrochloride in infusion fluids.

Ethanol

Nonproprietary Names BP : Ethanol (96%), JP: Ethanol, PhEur: Ethanolum (96 per centum), USP: Alcohol

Synonyms

Ethyl alcohol; ethyl hydroxide; grain alcohol; methyl carbinol.

Molecular Formula

C_2H_6O (46.07)

Characteristics

Alcohol is a clear, colorless, mobile, and volatile liquid with a slight, characteristic odor and burning taste.

Typical Properties

Boiling point : 78.15°C

Flammability : readily flammable, burning with a blue, smokeless flame.

Flash point : 14°C (closed cup)

Solubility : miscible with chloroform, ether, glycerin, and water (with rise of temperature and contraction of volume).

Pharmaceutical Applications

Ethanol and aqueous ethanol solutions of various concentrations are widely used in pharmaceutical formulations and cosmetics. Although ethanol is primarily used as a solvent it is also employed in solutions as an antimicrobial preservative. Topical ethanol solutions are also used as penetration enhancers and as disinfectants.

Stability and Storage Conditions

Aqueous ethanol solutions may be sterilized by autoclaving or by filtration and should be stored in airtight containers, in a cool place.

Incompatibilities

In acidic conditions, ethanol solutions may react vigorously with oxidizing materials. Mixtures with alkali may darken in color due to a reaction with residual amounts of aldehyde. Organic salts or acacia may be precipitated from aqueous solutions or dispersions. Ethanol solutions are also incompatible with aluminum containers and may interact with some drugs.

Kaolin

Nonproprietary Names BP : Heavy kaolin, JP: Kaolin, PhEur: Kaolinum ponderosum, USP: Kaolin

Synonyms

Argilla; bolus alba; china clay; kaolinite; porcelain clay; weisserton; white bole.

Molecular Formula

$Al_2H_4O_9Si_2$ (258.16)

Characteristics

Kaolin occurs as a white to grayish-white colored, unctuous powder free from gritty particles. It has a characteristic earthy or clay-like taste and when moistened with water, becomes darker in color and develops a clay-like odor.

Typical Properties

Acidity/alkalinity : pH = 4.0-7.5 for a 20% w/v aqueous slurry.

Hardness (Mohs) : 2.0, very low.

Solubility : practically insoluble in water, organic solvents, cold dilute acids, and solutions of alkali hydroxides.

Specific gravity : 2.6

Pharmaceutical Applications

Kaolin is a naturally occurring mineral used in oral and topical pharmaceutical formulations. It has been used as a suspending vehicle. In topical preparations, sterilized kaolin has been used in poultices and as a dusting powder. Therapeutically, kaolin has been used in oral antidiarrheal preparations

Stability and Storage Conditions

Kaolin is a stable material. Since it is a naturally occurring material, kaolin is commonly contaminated with microorganisms such as *Bacillus anthracis*, *Clostridium tetani,* and *Clostridium welchii*. However, kaolin may be sterilized by heating at a temperature greater than 160°C for not less than 1 hour.

Kaolin should be stored in a well-closed container in a cool, dry, place.

Incompatibilities

Drugs reportedly affected by kaolin include: amoxicillin; ampicillin; cimetidine; digoxin; lincomycin; phenytoin; and tetracycline. Warfarin absorption by rat intestine *in-vitro* was reported not to be affected by kaolin.

Colloidal Silica

Nonproprietary Names BP : Colloidal anhydrous silica, PhEur: Silica colloidalis, anhydrica, USP: Colloidal silicon dioxide

Synonyms

Aerosil; Cab-O-Sil; colloidal silica; fumed silica; light anhydrous silicic acid; silicic anhydride; silicon dioxide fumed; Wacker HDK.

Molecular Formula

SiO_2 (60.08)

Characteristics

Colloidal silicon dioxide is submicroscopic fumed silica with a particle size of about 15 nm. It is a light, loose, bluish-white colored, odorless, tasteless, nongritty amorphous powder.

Pharmaceutical Applications

Colloidal silicon dioxide is widely used in pharmaceuticals, cosmetics, and food products. Its small particle size and large specific surface area give it desirable flow characteristics which are exploited to improve the flow properties of dry powders in a number of processes, e.g., tableting.

In aerosols, other than those for inhalation, colloidal silicon dioxide is used to promote particulate suspension, eliminate hard settling and minimize the clogging of spray nozzles. Colloidal silicon dioxide is also used as a tablet disintegrant and as an adsorbent dispersing agent for liquids in powders or suppositories.

Stability and Storage Conditions

Colloidal silicon dioxide is hygroscopic, but adsorbs large quantities of water without liquefying. When used in aqueous systems at a pH between 0-7.5 colloidal silicon dioxide is effective in increasing the viscosity of a system. However, at a pH greater than 7.5 the viscosity-increasing properties of colloidal silicon dioxide are reduced and at a pH greater than 10.7 this ability is lost entirely since the silicon dioxide dissolves to form silicates. Colloidal silicon dioxide powder should be stored in a well-closed container.

Some grades of colloidal silicon dioxide have hydrophobic surface treatments, which greatly minimize its hygroscopicity.

Incompatibilities

Incompatible with diethylstilbestrol preparations

Magnesium carbonate

Nonproprietary Names BP : Heavy magnesium carbonate and, Light magnesium carbonate, JP: Magnesium carbonate, PhEur: Magnesii subcarbonas ponderosus and Magnesii subcarbonas levis, USP: Magnesium carbonate

Molecular Formula

Magnesium carbonate is not a homogeneous material but may consist of the rarely encountered anhydrous material, $MgCO_3$, the normal hydrate and the basic hydrate. Basic magnesium carbonate, probably the commonest form, may vary in formula between light magnesium carbonate, $(MgCO_3)_3 . Mg(OH)_2$.

$3H_2O$ and magnesium carbonate hydroxide, $(MgCO_3)_4.Mg(OH)_2.5H_2O$. Normal magnesium carbonate is a hydrous magnesium carbonate with a varying amount of water, $MgCO_3.xH_2O$. The molecular weights of the heavy and light forms of magnesium carbonate are 383.32 and 365.30 respectively.

Characteristics

Magnesium carbonate occurs as light, white-colored friable masses or as a bulky, white-colored powder. It has a slightly earthy taste and is odorless, but since it has a highly absorptive ability, magnesium carbonate can absorb odors.

Pharmaceutical Applications

As an excipient, magnesium carbonate is mainly used as a directly compressible tablet diluent in concentrations up to 45% w/w. Heavy magnesium carbonate produces tablets with high crushing strength, low friability, and good disintegration properties. It is also used to adsorb liquids, such as flavors, in tableting processes.

Magnesium carbonate is additionally used as a food additive and therapeutically as an antacid.

Stability and Storage Conditions

Magnesium carbonate is stable in dry air and on exposure to light. The bulk material should be stored in a well-closed container in a cool, dry, place.

Incompatibilities

Acids will dissolve magnesium carbonate, with the liberation of carbon dioxide. Slight alkalinity is imparted to water.

Starch

Nonproprietary Names BP : Maize starch, Potato starch, Rice starch, Tapioca starch, Wheat starch, JP: Corn starch, Rice starch, Potato starch, Wheat starch, PhEur: Maydis amylum (corn starch), Oryzae amylum (rice starch), Solani amylum (potato starch), Tritici amylum (wheat starch), USP: Starch

Synonyms

Amido; amidon; amilo; amylum; Aytex P; Fluftex W; Melojel; Paygel 55; Pure-Dent; Purity 21.

Molecular Formula

$(C_6H_{10}O_5)_n$

Where $n = 300\text{-}1000$.

Characteristics

Starch occurs as an odorless and tasteless, fine, white-colored powder comprised of very small spherical or ovoid granules whose size and shape are characteristic for each botanical variety.

Pharmaceutical Applications

Starch is used in topical preparations; for example, it is widely used in dusting powders for its absorbency, and is used as a protective covering in ointment formulations applied to the skin. Starch mucilage has also been applied to the skin as an emollient, has formed the base of some enemas, and has been used in the treatment of iodine poisoning.

Starch is also used as an excipient primarily in oral solid-dosage formulations where, it is utilized as a binder, diluents and disintegrates.

Therapeutically, rice starch-based solutions have been used in the prevention and treatment of dehydration due to acute diarroheal diseases.

Stability and Storage Conditions

Dry, unheated starch is stable if protected from high humidity. When used as a diluent or disintegrant in solid-dosage forms, starch is considered to be inert under normal storage conditions. However, heated starch solutions or pastes are physically unstable and are readily attacked by microorganisms to form a wide variety of starch derivatives and modified starches, which have unique physical properties.

Starch should be stored in an airtight container in a cool, dry, place.

Zinc Stearate

Nonproprietary Names BP : Zinc stearate, PhEur: Zinci stearas, USP: Zinc stearate

Synonyms

Stearic acid zinc salt; zinc distearate.

Molecular Formula

$C_{36}H_{70}O_4Zn$ (632.33)

Characteristics

Zinc stearate occurs as a fine, white, bulky, hydrophobic powder, free from grittiness and with a faint characteristic odor.

Typical Properties

Auto ignition temperature : 421°C

Density (true) : 1.09 g/cm^3

Density (tapped) : 0.26 g/cm^3 for standard grade (Durham Chemicals).

Flash point : 277°C

Melting point : 120-122°C

Solubility : practically insoluble in ethanol (95%), ether, and water; soluble in benzene.

Pharmaceutical Applications

It is used as a thickening and opacifying agent in cosmetic and pharmaceutical creams and as a dusting powder. Zinc stearate is primarily used in pharmaceutical formulations as a lubricant in tablet and capsule manufacture at concentrations up to 1.5% w/w.

Stability and Storage Conditions

Zinc stearate is stable and should be stored in a well-closed container in a cool, dry, place.

Incompatibilities

Zinc stearate is decomposed by dilute acids.

Calcium Carbonate

Nonproprietary Names BP : Calcium carbonate, JP: Calcium carbonate, PhEur: Calcii carbonas, USP: Calcium carbonate; carbonic acid, calcium salt (1:1); calcium carbonate (1:1).

Synonyms

Cal-Carb; creta preparada; E170; Millicarb; Pharma-Carb; precipitated calcium carbonate; precipitated carbonate of lime; precipitated chalk; Sturcal.

Molecular Formula

$CaCO_3$ (100.09)

Characteristics

Calcium carbonate occurs as an odorless and tasteless white powder or crystals.

Pharmaceutical Applications

It is used as a base for medicated dental preparations, and as a buffering and dissolution aid in dispersible tablets. Calcium carbonate, employed as a pharmaceutical excipient, is mainly used in solid-dosage forms as a diluent.

Calcium carbonate is used as a bulking agent in tablet sugar- coating processes and as an opacifier in tablet film coating.

Calcium carbonate is also used as a food additive and therapeutically as an antacid and calcium supplement.

Stability and Storage Conditions

Calcium carbonate is stable and should be stored in a well-closed container in a cool, dry place.

Incompatibilities

Incompatible with acids and ammonium salts

Sodium Alginate

Nonproprietary Names BP : Sodium alginate, PhEur: Natrii alginas, USP: Sodium alginate

Synonyms

Algin; alginic acid, sodium salt; E401; Kelcosol; Keltone; Manucol; Manugel; Pronova; Protanal; Satialgine-H8; sodium polymannuronate.

Molecular Formula

Sodium alginate consists chiefly of the sodium salt of alginic acid, which is a mixture of polyuronic acids composed of residues of D-mannuronic acid and L-guluronic acid.

The block structure and molecular weight of sodium alginate samples has been investigated.

Characteristics

Sodium alginate occurs as an odorless and tasteless, white to pale yellowish-brown colored powder.

Pharmaceutical Applications

Sodium alginate is used in a variety of oral and topical pharmaceutical formulations. In tablet formulations, sodium alginate may be used as both a binder and disintegrant; it has been used as a diluent in capsule formulations. Sodium alginate has also been used in the preparation of sustained- release oral formulations since it can delay the dissolution of a drug from tablets, capsules, and aqueous suspensions.

In topical formulations, sodium alginate is widely used as a thickening and suspending agent in a variety of pastes, creams, and gels, and as a stabilizing agent for oil-in-water emulsions.

Sodium alginate is also used in cosmetics and food products.

Stability and Storage Conditions

Sodium alginate is a hygroscopic material although it is stable if stored at low relative humidities and a cool temperature.

Aqueous solutions of sodium alginate are most stable between pH 4-10; below pH 3, alginic acid is precipitated. A 1% w/v aqueous solution of sodium alginate exposed to differing temperatures had a viscosity 60-80% its original value after storage for 2 years. Solutions should not be stored in metal containers.

The bulk material should be stored in an airtight container in a cool, dry, place.

Incompatibilities

Sodium alginate is incompatible with acridine derivatives, crystal violet, phenylmercuric acetate and nitrate, calcium salts, heavy metals, and ethanol in concentrations greater than 5%. Low concentrations of electrolytes cause an increase in viscosity but high electrolyte concentrations cause salting-out of sodium alginate; salting-out occurs if more than 4% of sodium chloride is present.

Carboxymethylcellulose

Nonproprietary Names BP : Carmellose sodium, JP: Carmellose sodium, PhEur: Carboxymethylcellulosum natricum, USP: Carboxymethylcellulose sodium

Synonyms

Akucell; Aquasorb; Blanose; Cekol; cellulose gum; CMC sodium; Finnfix; Nymcel; sodium carboxymethylcellulose; sodium cellulose glycolate; sodium CMC; Tylose CB.

Molecular Formula

The USP describes carboxymethylcellulose sodium as the sodium salt of a polycarboxymethyl ether of cellulose. Typical molecular weight is 90 000-700 000.

Characteristics

Carboxymethylcellulose sodium occurs as a white to almost white colored, odorless, granular powder.

Pharmaceutical Applications

Carboxymethylcellulose sodium is widely used in oral and topical pharmaceutical formulations primarily for its viscosity-increasing properties.

Viscous aqueous solutions are used to suspend powders intended for either topical application or oral and parenteral administration. Carboxymethylcellulose sodium may also be used as a tablet binder and disintegrant, and to stabilize emulsions.

Higher concentrations, usually 3-6%, of the medium viscosity grade is used to produce gels which can be used as the base for applications and pastes; glycols are often included in such gels to prevent drying out. Carboxymethylcellulose sodium is additionally one of the main ingredients of self-adhesive ostomy, wound care, and dermatological patches where it is used to absorb wound exudate or transepidermal water and sweat. Carboxymethylcellulose sodium is also used in cosmetics, toiletries, incontinence, personal hygiene, and food products.

Stability and Storage Conditions

Carboxymethylcellulose sodium is a stable, though hygroscopic material. Under high humidity conditions carboxymethylcellulose sodium can absorb a large quantity (> 50%) of water. In tablets, this has been associated with a decrease in tablet hardness and an increase in disintegration time.

Aqueous solutions are stable between pH 2-10; below pH 2 precipitation can occur while above pH 10 solution viscosity rapidly decreases. Generally, solutions exhibit maximum viscosity and stability at pH 7-9.

The bulk material should be stored in a well-closed container in a cool, dry, place.

Incompatibilities

Carboxymethylcellulose sodium is incompatible with strongly acidic solutions and with the soluble salts of iron and some other metals, such as aluminum, mercury, and zinc. Precipitation can occur at pH < 2 and when mixed with ethanol (95%).

Phenol

Nonproprietary Names BP : Phenol, JP: Phenol, PhEur: Phenolum, USP: Phenol

Synonyms

Carbolic acid; hydroxybenzene; oxybenzene; phenic acid; phenyl hydrate; phenyl hydroxide; phenylic acid; phenylic alcohol.

Molecular Formula

C_6H_6O (94.11)

Characteristics

Phenol occurs as colorless to light pink, caustic, deliquescent needle-shaped crystals or crystalline masses with a characteristic odor. When heated gently phenol melts forming a highly refractive liquid.

Typical Properties

Autoignition temperature : 715°C

Boiling point : 181.8°C

Density : 1.071 g/cm^3

Dissociation constant : pK_a = 10 at 25°C

Flash point : 79°C (closed cup)

Explosive limits : 2% lower limit; 9% upper limit.

Freezing point : 40.9°C

Melting point : 43°C

Solubility :

Solvent	Solubility at 20 °C
Carbon disulfide	Very soluble
Chloroform	Very soluble
Ethanol (95%)	Very soluble
Ether	Very soluble
Fixed oils	Very soluble
Glycerin	Very soluble
Mineral oil	1 in 70
Volatile oils	Very soluble
Water	1 in 15

Pharmaceutical Applications

Phenol is used mainly as an antimicrobial preservative in parenteral pharmaceutical products although it has also been used in topical pharmaceutical formulations and cosmetics. It should not be used to preserve preparations that are to be freeze-dried Phenol is also widely used as an antiseptic, disinfectant, and therapeutic agent.

Stability and Storage Conditions

When exposed to air and light, phenol turns a red or brown color, the color being influenced by the presence of metallic impurities. Oxidizing agents also hasten the color change. Aqueous solutions of phenol are stable. Oily solutions for injection may be sterilized in hermetically sealed containers by dry heat. The bulk material should be stored in a well- closed container at a temperature not exceeding 15°C.

Incompatibilities

Phenol undergoes a number of chemical reactions characteristic of alcohols; however, it possesses a tautomeric enol structure that is weakly acidic. It will form salts with sodium hydroxide or potassium hydroxide, but not with their carbonates or bicarbonates. Phenol is a reducing agent and is capable of reacting with ferric salts in neutral to acidic solutions to form a greenish-colored complex. Phenol decolorizes dilute iodine solutions, forming hydrogen iodide and iodophenol; stronger solutions of iodine react with phenol to form the insoluble 2,4,6-triiodophenol.

Phenol is incompatible with albumin and gelatin since they are precipitated. It forms a liquid or soft mass when triturated with some compounds, e.g., camphor, menthol, thymol, acetaminophen, phenacetin, chloral hydrate, phenazone, ethyl aminobenzoate, methenamine, phenyl salicylate, resorcinol, terpin hydrate, sodium phosphate, or other eutectic formers. Phenol also softens cocoa butter in suppository mixtures.

Tricalcium phosphate

Nonproprietary Names BP : Calcium phosphate, PhEur: Tricalcii phosphate, USP: Tribasic calcium phosphate

Synonyms

Calcium orthophosphate; hydroxyapatite; phosphoric acid calcium salt (2:3); precipitated calcium phosphate; tertiary calcium phosphate; Tri-Cafos; tricalcium diorthophosphate.

Molecular Formula

$Ca_3(PO_4)_2$ (310.20)

$Ca_5(OH)(PO_4)_3$ (502.32)

Characteristics

Tribasic calcium phosphate is a white, amorphous, odorless, and tasteless powder.

Typical Properties

Acidity/alkalinity : pH = 6.8 (20% slurry of *TRI-TAB*)

Density : 3.14 g/cm^3

Density (bulk) : 0.80 g/cm^3

Density (tapped) : 0.95 g/cm^3

Flowability : 24.6 g/s

Melting point : 1670°C

Particle size distribution :

Solubility : soluble in dilute mineral acids; very slightly soluble in water; practically insoluble in acetic acid and alcohols.

Pharmaceutical Applications

Tribasic calcium phosphate is widely used as a tablet and capsule diluent in either direct compression or wet-granulation processes. As with dibasic calcium phosphate, a lubricant and a disintegrant should be incorporated in capsule or tablet formulations, which include tribasic calcium phosphate. Tribasic calcium phosphate is most widely used in vitamin and mineral preparations as a diluent and calcium source but may also be used in some applications as a disintegrant.

Tribasic calcium phosphate is also widely used in food applications as an anticaking agent.

Stability and Storage Conditions

Tribasic calcium phosphate is a stable material and is not liable to cake. The bulk material should be stored in a well-closed container in a cool, dry, place.

Incompatibilities

Calcium salts are incompatible with tetracycline antibiotics. Tribasic calcium phosphate is also incompatible with tocopheryl acetate (but not tocopheryl succinate). It influences the absorption of vitamin D and may form sparingly soluble phosphates with hormones.

Sodium lauryl sulphate

Nonproprietary Names BP : Sodium lauryl sulfate, JP: Sodium lauryl sulfate, PhEur: Natrii laurilsulfas, USP: Sodium lauryl sulfate

Synonyms

Dodecyl sodium sulfate; Elfan 240; Empicol LZ; Maprofix 563; Nutrapon W; sodium dodecyl sulfate; sodium laurilsulfate; sodium monododecyl sulfate; sodium monolauryl sulfate; Stepanol WA 100.

Molecular Formula

$C_{12}H_{25}NaO_4S$ (288.38)

Characteristics

Sodium lauryl sulfate consists of white or cream to pale yellow-colored crystals, flakes or powder having a smooth feel, a soapy, bitter taste and a faint odor of fatty substances.

Typical Properties

Acidity/alkalinity : pH = 7.0-9.5 (1% w/v aqueous solution).

Acid value : 0

Critical micelle concentration : 8.2 mmol/L (0.23 g/L) at 20°C.

Density : 1.07 g/cm^3 at 20°C

Melting point : 204-207°C (for pure substance).

Solubility : freely soluble in water, giving an opalescent solution; practically insoluble in chloroform and ether.

Pharmaceutical Applications

Sodium lauryl sulfate is an anionic surfactant employed in a wide range of nonparenteral pharmaceutical formulations and cosmetics. It is a detergent and wetting agent effective in both alkaline and acidic conditions. In recent years it has found application in analytical electrophoretic techniques: SDS (sodium lauryl sulfate) polyacrylamide gel electrophoresis is one or the more widely used techniques for the analysis of proteins; and sodium lauryl sulfate has been used to enhance the selectivity of micellar electrokinetic chromatography (MEKC).

Stability and Storage Conditions

Sodium lauryl sulfate is stable under normal storage conditions. However, in solution, under extreme conditions, i.e., pH 2.5 or below, it undergoes hydrolysis to lauryl alcohol and sodium bisulfate.

The bulk material should be stored in a well-closed container away from strong oxidizing agents in a cool, dry, place.

Incompatibilities

Sodium lauryl sulfate reacts with cationic surfactants causing loss of activity even in concentrations too low to cause precipitation. Unlike soaps, it is compatible with dilute acids and calcium and magnesium ions.

Solutions of sodium lauryl sulfate (pH 9.5-10.0) are mildly corrosive to mild steel, copper, brass, bronze, and aluminum. Sodium lauryl sulfate is also incompatible with some alkaloidal salts and precipitates with lead and potassium salts.

Saccharin sodium

Nonproprietary Names BP : Saccharin sodium, JP: Saccharin sodium, PhEur: Saccharinum natricum, USP: Saccharin sodium

Synonyms

1,2-Benzisothiazolin-3-one 1,1-dioxide, sodium salt; Britsol; Crystallose; Dagutan; Kristallose; sodium o-benzosulfimide; soluble gluside; soluble saccharin; Sucaryl; Sucromat; Syncal S.

Molecular Formula

$C_7H_4NNaO_3S$	205.16
$C_7H_4NNaO_3S.OH_2O$ (84%)	217.24
$C_7H_4NNaO_3S.2H_2O$ (76%)	241.19

Characteristics

Saccharin sodium occurs as a white, odorless or faintly aromatic, efflorescent, crystalline powder. It has an intensely sweet taste, with a metallic aftertaste, which at normal levels of use can be detected by approximately 25% of the population. Saccharin sodium can contain variable amounts of water.

Typical Properties

Acidity/alkalinity : pH = 6.6 (10% w/v aqueous solution)

Density (bulk) : 0.8-1.1 g/cm^3 (76% saccharin sodium); 0.86 g/cm^3 (84% saccharin sodium).

Density (particle) : 1.70 g/cm^3 (84% saccharin sodium)

Density (tapped) : 0.9-1.2 g/cm^3 (76% saccharin sodium); 0.96 g/cm^3 (84% saccharin sodium).

Melting point : decomposes upon heating.

Solubility :

Solvent	Solubility at 25 °C Unless otherwise stated
Buffer solutions :	
pH 2.2 (phthalate)	1 in 1.15
	1 in 0.66 at 60 °C
pH 4.0 (citrate-phosphate)	1 in 1.21
	1 in 0.69 at 60 °C
pH 7.0 (citrate-phosphate)	1 in 1.21
	1 in 0.66 at 60 °C
pH 9.0 (borate)	1 in 1.21
	1 in 0.69 at 60 °C
Ethanol	1 in 102
Ethanol (95%)	1 in 50
Propylene glycol	1 in 3.5
Propan-2-ol	Practically insoluble
Water	1 in 1.2

Pharmaceutical Applications

Saccharin sodium is an intense sweetening agent used in beverages, food products, table-top sweeteners, and pharmaceutical formulations such as tablets, powders, medicated confectionery, gels, suspensions, and liquids. It is also used in vitamin preparations.

Saccharin sodium is considerably more soluble in water than saccharin and is also more frequently used in pharmaceutical formulations. Sweetening power is approximately 300 times that of sucrose. Saccharin sodium enhances flavor systems and may be used to mask some unpleasant taste characteristics.

Stability and Storage Conditions

Saccharin sodium is stable under the normal range of conditions employed in formulations. It is only when exposed to a high temperature (125°C) at a low pH (pH 2) for over 1 hour that significant decomposition occurs. The 84% grade is the most stable form of saccharin sodium since the 76% form will dry further under ambient conditions.

Saccharin sodium should be stored in a well-closed container in a cool, dry, place.

Cetostearyl Alcohol

Nonproprietary Names BP : Cetostearyl alcohol, PhEur: Alcohol cetylicus et stearylicus, USP: Cetostearyl alcohol, CTFA: Cetearyl alcohol

Synonyms

Cetearyl alcohol.

Molecular Formula

Cetostearyl alcohol is a mixture of solid aliphatic alcohols consisting mainly of stearyl ($C_{18}H_{38}O$) and cetyl ($C_{16}H_{34}O$) alcohols. The proportion of stearyl to cetyl alcohol varies considerably but usually consists of about 50-70% stearyl alcohol and 20-35% cetyl alcohol, with limits specified in pharmacopeias.

Characteristics

Cetostearyl alcohol occurs as white or cream-colored unctuous masses, or almost white-colored flakes or granules. It has a faint characteristic sweet odor. On heating, cetostearyl alcohol melts to a clear, colorless, or pale yellow-colored liquid free of suspended matter.

Pharmaceutical Applications

Cetostearyl alcohol is used in cosmetics and topical pharmaceuticals. In topical pharmaceutical formulations cetostearyl alcohol will increase the viscosity and impart body in both water-in-oil and oil-in-water emulsions. Cetostearyl alcohol will stablize an emulsion and also act as a co-emulsifier, thus decreasing the amount of surfactant required to from a stable emulsion. Cetostearyl alcohol is also used in the preparation of nonaqueous creams and sticks.

Stability and Storage Conditions

Cetostearyl alcohol is stable under normal storage conditions. Cetostearyl alcohol should be stored in a well-closed container in a cool, dry, place.

Incompatibilities

Incompatible with strong oxidizing agents and metal salts.

Carnauba Wax

Nonproprietary Names BP : Carnauba wax, JP: Carnauba wax, PhEur: Cera carnauba, USP: Carnauba wax

Synonyms

Brazil wax; caranda wax.

Molecular Formula

Carnauba wax consists primarily of a complex mixture of esters of acids and hydroxyacids. Also present are acids, oxypolyhydric alcohols, hydrocarbons, resinous matter, and water.

Characteristics

Carnauba wax occurs as a light brown to pale yellow-colored powder, flakes, or irregular lumps of a hard, brittle wax. It possesses a characteristic bland odor and practically no taste. It is free from rancidity. Commercially, various types and grades are available.

Typical Properties

Flash point : 270-330°C

Refractive index : n_D^{90} = 1.450

Solubility : soluble in warm chloroform, and warm toluene; slightly soluble in boiling ethanol (95%); practically insoluble in water.

Specific gravity : 0.990-0.999 at 25°C

Unsaponified matter : 50-55%

Pharmaceutical Applications

Carnauba wax is widely used in cosmetics, certain foods, and pharmaceutical formulations.

Carnauba wax is the hardest and highest melting of the waxes commonly used in pharmaceutical formulations and is used primarily as a 10% w/v aqueous emulsion to polish sugar coated tablets. Aqueous emulsions may be prepared by mixing carnauba wax with an ethanolamine compound and oleic acid. The carnauba wax coating produces tablets of good luster without rubbing. Carnauba wax may also be used in powder form to polish sugar coated tablets.

Stability and Storage Conditions

Carnauba wax is stable and should be stored in a well-closed container, in a cool, dry, place.

Butylated Hydroxytoluene

Nonproprietary Names BP : Butylated hydroxytoluene, PhEur: Butylhydroxytoluenum, USP: Butylated hydroxytoluene

Synonyms

Advastab-401; Agidol; Annulex BHT; Antioxidant 30; Antrancine 8; BHT; 2,6-bis(1,1-dimethylethyl)-4-methylphenol; butylhydroxytoluene; Dalpac; dibutylated hydroxytoluene; 2,6-di- tert-butyl-p-cresol; 3,5-di-tert-butyl-4-hydroxytoluene.

Molecular Formula

$C_{15}H_{24}O$ (220.35)

Characteristics

Butylated hydroxytoluene occurs as a white or pale yellow crystalline solid or powder with a faint characteristic odor.

Typical Properties

Boiling point : 265°C

Density (bulk) : 0.48-0.60 g/cm^3, Density (true): 1.031 g/cm^3,

Flash point : 127°C (open cup)

Latent heat of fusion : 23.4 J/g (16.5 cal/g)

Melting point : 70°C

Partition coefficient : Octanol: water = 4.17-5.80

Solubility : practically insoluble in water, glycerin, propylene glycol, solutions of alkali hydroxides, and dilute aqueous mineral acids. Freely soluble in acetone, benzene, ethanol (95%), ether, methanol, toluene, fixed oils, and mineral oil. More soluble in food oils and fats than butylated hydroxyanisole.

Pharmaceutical Applications

Butylated hydroxytoluene is used as an antioxidant in cosmetics, foods, and pharmaceuticals. It is mainly used to delay or prevent oxidative rancidity of fats and oils and to prevent loss of activity of oil-soluble vitamins. Butylated hydroxytoluene is also used at 0.5-1% concentration in natural or synthetic rubber to provide enhanced color stability.

Butylated hydroxytoluene has some antiviral activity and has been used therapeutically to treat herpes simplex labialis.

Antioxidant use	Concentration (%)
Beta-Carotene	0.01
Edible vegetable oils	0.01
Essential oils and flavoring agents	0.02-0.5
Fats and oils	0.02
Fish oils	0.01-0.1
Inhalations	0.01
IM injections	0.03
IV injections	0.0009-0.002
Topical formulations	0.0075-0.1
Vitamin A	10 mg per million units

Stability and Storage Conditions

Exposure to light, moisture, and heat cause discoloration and a loss of activity. Butylated hydroxytoluene should be stored in a well-closed container, protected from light, in a cool, dry, place.

Incompatibilities

Butylated hydroxytoluene is phenolic and undergoes reactions characteristic of phenols. It is incompatible with strong oxidizing agents such as peroxides and permanganates. Contact with oxidizing agents may cause spontaneous combustion. Iron salts cause discoloration with loss of activity. Heating with catalytic amounts of acids causes rapid decomposition with the release of the flammable gas isobutylene.

Petrolatum

Nonproprietary Names BP : Yellow soft paraffin, JP: Yellow petrolatum, USP: Petrolatum

Synonyms

Mineral jelly; petroleum jelly; Snow white; Soft white; vaselinum flavum; yellow petrolatum; yellow petroleum jelly.

Molecular Formula

Petrolatum is a purified mixture of semisolid saturated hydrocarbons having the general formula C_nH_{2n+2}, and is obtained from petroleum. The hydrocarbons consist mainly of branched and unbranched chains although some cyclic alkanes and aromatic molecules with paraffin side chains may also be present.

Characteristics

Petrolatum is a pale yellow-to-yellow colored, translucent, soft unctuous mass. It is odorless, tasteless, and not more than slightly fluorescent by daylight, even when melted.

Pharmaceutical Applications

Petrolatum is mainly used in topical pharmaceutical formulations as an emollient-ointment base and it is poorly absorbed by the skin. Petrolatum is also used in creams and transdermal formulations and as an ingredient in lubricant formulations for medicated confectionery together with mineral oil.

Therapeutically, sterile gauze dressings containing petrolatum may be used for nonadherent wound dressings or as a packing material. Petrolatum is additionally widely used in cosmetics and in some food applications.

Use	Concentration (%)
Emollient topical creams	10-30
Topical emulsions	4-25
Topical ointments	Up to 100

Stability and Storage Conditions

Petrolatum is an inherently stable material due to the unreactive nature of its hydrocarbon components; most stability problems occur due to the presence of small quantities of impurities. On exposure to light these impurities may be oxidized to discolor the petrolatum and produce an undesirable odor. The extent of the oxidation varies depending upon the source of the petrolatum and the degree of refinement. Oxidation may be inhibited by the inclusion of a suitable antioxidant such as butylated hydroxyanisole, butylated hydroxytoluene, or alpha tocopherol.

Petrolatum should be stored in a well-closed container, protected from light, in a cool, dry, place.

Incompatibilities

Petrolatum is an inert material with few incompatibilities.

Isopropyl alcohol

Nonproprietary Names BP : Isopropyl alcohol, JP: Isopropanol, PhEur: Alcohol isopropylicus, USP: Isopropyl alcohol

Synonyms

Dimethyl carbinol; IPA; isopropanol; petrohol; 2-propanol; *sec*-propyl alcohol.

Molecular Formula

C_3H_8O (60.1)

Characteristics

Isopropyl alcohol is a clear, colorless, mobile, volatile, flammable liquid with a characteristic, spirituous odor resembling that of a mixture of ethanol and acetone; it has a slightly bitter taste.

Typical Properties

Autoignition temperature : 425°C

Boiling point : 82.4°C

Dielectric constant : D^{20} = 18.62

Explosive limits : 2.5-12.0% v/v in air.

Flammability : flammable.

Flash point : 11.7°C (closed cup); 13°C (open cup). The water azeotrope has a flash point of 16°C.

Freezing point : −89.5°C

Solubility : miscible with benzene, chloroform, ethanol, ether, glycerin, and water. Soluble in acetone; insoluble in salt solutions. Forms an azeotrope with water, containing 87.4% w/w isopropyl alcohol (boiling point = 80.37°C).

Pharmaceutical Applications

Isopropyl alcohol (propan-2-ol) is used in cosmetics and pharmaceutical formulations primarily as a solvent in topical formulations. It is not recommended for oral use due to its toxicity.

Although used in lotions, the marked degreasing properties of isopropyl alcohol may limit its usefulness in preparations used repeatedly. Isopropyl alcohol is also used as a solvent both for tablet film-coating and tablet granulation where the isopropyl alcohol is subsequently removed by evaporation.

Isopropyl alcohol has some antimicrobial activity and a 70% v/v aqueous solution is used as a topical disinfectant.

Stability and Storage Conditions

Isopropyl alcohol should be stored in an airtight container in a cool, dry, place.

Incompatibilities

Incompatible with oxidizing agents such as hydrogen peroxide and nitric acid, which cause decomposition. Isopropyl alcohol may be salted out from aqueous mixtures by the addition of sodium chloride, sodium sulfate, and other salts, or by the addition of sodium hydroxide.

Benzoic acid

Nonproprietary Names BP : Benzoic acid, JP: Benzoic acid, PhEur: Acidum benzoicum

USP : Benzoic acid

Synonyms

Benzenecarboxylic acid; benzeneformic acid; carboxybenzene; dracylic acid; phenylcarboxylic acid; phenylformic acid.

Molecular Formula

$C_7H_6O_2$ (122.12)

Characteristics

Benzoic acid occurs as feathery, light, white or colorless crystals or powder. It is essentially tasteless and odorless or with a slight characteristic odor suggestive of benzoin.

Typical Properties

Acidity/alkalinity : pH = 2.8 (saturated aqueous solution at 25°C)

Autoignition temperature : 570°C

Boiling point : 249.2°C

Density : 1.311 g/cm^3 for solid at 24°C; 1.075 g/cm^3 for liquid at 130°C.

Flash point : 121-131°C, Melting point: 122°C (begins to sublime at 100°C).

Partition coefficients : Benzene: water = 0.0044; Cyclohexane: water = 0.30;

Octanol : water = 1.87.

Solubility : apparent aqueous solubility of benzoic acid may be enhanced by the addition of citric acid or sodium acetate to the solution.

Solvent	Solubility at 25 °C unless otherwise stated
Acetone	1 in 2.3
Benzene	1 in 9.4
Carbon disulfide	1 in 30
Carbon tetrachloride	1 in 15.2
Chloroform	1 in 4.5
Cyclohexane	1 in 14.6
Ethanol	1 in 2.7 at 15 °C
	1 in 2.2
Ethanol (76%)	1 in 3.72
Ethanol (54%)	1 in 6.27
Ethanol (25%)	1 in 68
Ether	1 in 3
Fixed oils	Freely soluble
Methanol	1 in 1.8
Toluene	1 in 11
Water	1 in 300

Stability and Storage Conditions

Aqueous solutions of benzoic acid may be sterilized by autoclaving or by filtration.

A 0.1% w/v aqueous solution of benzoic acid has been reported as being stable for at least 8 weeks when stored in polyvinyl chloride bottles, at room temperature.

When added to a suspension benzoic acid dissociates with the benzoate anion adsorbing onto the suspended drug particles. This adsorption alters the charge at the surface of the particles which may in turn affect the physical stability of the suspension.

The bulk material should be stored in a well-closed container in a cool, dry, place.

Incompatibilities

Undergoes typical reactions of an organic acid, e.g., with alkalis or heavy metals. Preservative activity may be reduced by interaction with kaolin.

Menthol

Nonproprietary Names BP : Racementhol, JP: *dl*-Menthol, PhEur: Mentholum racemicum, USP: Menthol

Synonyms

Hexahydrothymol; 2-isopropyl-5-methylcyclohexanol; 4-isopropyl-1-methylcyclohexan-3-ol; 3-*p*-menthanol; *p*-menthan- 3-ol; *dl*-menthol; peppermint camphor; racemic menthol.

Molecular Formula

$C_{10}H_{20}O$ (156.27)

Characteristics

Racemic menthol is a mixture of equal parts of the (1*R*,2*S*,5*R*)- and (1*S*,2*R*,5*S*)-isomers of menthol. It is a free flowing or agglomerated crystalline powder or colorless, prismatic or acicular shiny crystals, with a strong characteristic odor and taste. The crystalline form may change with time due to sublimation within a closed vessel. The USP specifies that menthol may be either naturally occurring *l*-menthol or synthetically prepared racemic or *l*-menthol. However, the JP and PhEur, along with other pharmacopeias, include two separate monographs for racemic and *l*- menthol.

Typical Properties

Boiling point : 212°C

Flash point : 93°C

Melting point : 34-36°C

Refractive index : n_D^{20} = 1.4615

Solubility : very soluble in ethanol (95%), chloroform, and ether; very slightly soluble in glycerin; practically insoluble in water.

Pharmaceutical Applications

Menthol is widely used in pharmaceuticals, confectionery, and toiletry products as a flavoring agent or odor enhancer. In addition to its characteristic peppermint flavor, *l*-menthol, which occurs naturally, also exerts a cooling or refreshing sensation which is exploited in many topical preparations. Unlike mannitol, which exerts a similar effect due to a negative heat of solution, *l*-menthol interacts directly with the body's coldness receptors. *d*-Menthol has no cooling effect, while racemic menthol imparts an effect approximately half that of menthol.

When used to flavor tablets menthol is generally dissolved in ethanol (95%) and sprayed on tablet granules and not used as a solid excipient.

Menthol has been investigated as a skin-penetration enhancer and is also used in perfumery, tobacco products, and as a therapeutic agent.

Use	Concentration (%)
Pharmaceutical products	
Inhalation	0.02-0.05
Oral suspension	0.003
Oral syrup	0.005-0.015
Tablets	0.2-0.4
Topical formulations	0.05-10.0
Cosmetic products	
Toothpaste	0.4
Mouthwash	0.1-2.0
Oral spray	0.3

Stability and Storage Conditions

A formulation containing menthol 1% w/w in aqueous cream has been reported to be stable for up to 18 months when stored at room temperature. Menthol should be stored in a well-closed container at a temperature not exceeding 25°C, since it sublimes readily.

Incompatibilities

Incompatible with butylchloral hydrate, camphor, chloral hydrate, chromium trioxide, phenol, potassium permanganate, pyrogallol, resorcinol, and thymol.

Magnesium stearate

Nonproprietary Names BP : Magnesium stearate, JP: Magnesium stearate, PhEur: Magnesii stearas, USP: Magnesium stearate

Synonyms

Magnesium octadecanoate; stearic acid magnesium salt; octadecanoic acid, magnesium salt.

Molecular Formula

$C_{36}H_{70}MgO_4$ (591.34)

Characteristics

Crystalline forms: high purity magnesium stearate has been isolated as a trihydrate, a dihydrate, and an anhydrate.

Typical Properties

Density (bulk): 0.159 g/cm^3

Density (tapped) : 0.286 g/cm^3

Density (true) : 1.092 g/cm^3

Flash point : 250°C

Flowability : poorly flowing, cohesive powder.

Solubility : practically insoluble in ethanol, ethanol (95%), ether and water; slightly soluble in warm benzene and warm ethanol (95%).

Pharmaceutical Applications

Magnesium stearate is widely used in cosmetics, foods, and pharmaceutical formulations. It is primarily used as a lubricant in capsule and tablet manufacture at concentrations between 0.25-5.0%. It is also used in barrier creams.

Stability and Storage Conditions

Magnesium stearate is stable and should be stored in a well-closed container in a cool, dry place.

Incompatibilities

Incompatible with strong acids, alkalis and iron salts. Avoid mixing with strong oxidizing materials. Magnesium stearate cannot be used in products containing aspirin, some vitamins, and most alkaloidal salts.

Some Newer Exicipients Used In cosmetics

The addition of proteins in cosmetic has been considerably increased in recent decades. And if such proteins are derived from vegetable sources it is then considered more safer and effective. High-protein plants most commonly used as starting material for producing vegetable proteins are wheat and corn gluten, soy, rice and oat protein concentrates, and defatted oilseeds (peanuts, almond, sunflower). Among the large variety of vegetable proteins wheat gluten and soy globulins are by far of the widest use and interest. Wheat gluten (commonly known as wheat protein) is a unique cereal protein of high elasticity when hydrated. Soy proteins are useful due to their gelling and emulsifying effects.And also have remarkable collagen and elastin synthesizing property.

Formulating Proteins In cosmetics

Soluble proteins are suitable to be incorporated in almost all common forms as emulsions, lotions, gels, and powders. The table below gives a brief overview about the use of proteins and their derivatives in skin and hair care preparations.

A. Proteins in Skin Care Products

1. **Protein Hydrolysates**

   Example: hydrolyzed collagen/elastin/silk/wheat

   Function: humectant, film former, conditioner

   Use: 0.2 - 5% in creams, lotions

2. **Highly Water-Soluble Proteins**

   Example: desamido collagen, serum albumin

   Function: humectant, protectant, conditioner

   Use: 0.01 - 0.1% in creams, lotions

3. **Gelatin**

   Function: thickener, film former, emulsion stabilizer.

   Use: 1 - 2% in emulsions

4. **Protein Condensates**

   Example: potassium cocoyl hydrolyzed collagen

   Function: co-emulsifier

   Use: 0.5 - 2% in O/W emulsions

5. **Insoluble Proteins**

   Example: silk powder, insoluble keratin/elastin

   Function: oil absorbent, cohesive agent

   Use: 1 - 5% in powder makeup preparations

B. Proteins in Hair Care Products

1. **Protein Hydrolysates**

   Example: hydrolyzed collagen/keratin/silk/wheat

   Function: conditioner, buffering agent

   Use: 0.2 - 2% in shampoos, conditioners, rinses

2. **Protein Condensates**

   Example: hydrolyzed wheat protein polysiloxane copolymer, AMP-isostearoyl hydrolyzed collagen, alkyldimonium hydroxy -propyl   hydrolyzed elastin

Function: conditioner

Use: 0.05 - 3% in conditioners, relaxers, rinses

3. Soluble Proteins

Example: soluble keratin, soluble wheat protein

Function: permanent conditioner

Use: 0.5 - 5% in conditioning perms

4. Special Protein Condensates

Example: potassium undecylenoyl hydrolyzed collagen, potassium abietoyl hydrolyzed collagen

Function: anti-dandruff

Use: 0.5 - 2% in shampoos

Some Examples

1. Hydrolyzed Corn and Hydrolyzed Soy Protein

The proteins of corn and soy may be combined and hydrolyzed with enzyme under mild conditions for several hours until the target molecular weight is achieved. The resultant hydrolyzed proteins may then be concentrated.

2. Hydrolyzed Silk

Hydrolyzed silk has been reported to be prepared from the cocoon of the silkworm moth (*Bombyx mori*). The silk thread is isolated from the cocoon and the fibers are cleaned and degummed. The individual silk fiber is then wound with other silk fibers to create one long thread. The threads are then combed to remove noils, which are short fibers considered to be by-products of the textile industry. The noils are used in the production of hydrolyzed silk proteins through carefully controlled hydrolysis.The resultant material is a 5% solution of a water soluble silk protein.

3. Hydrolyzed Serum Protein

Hydrolyzed serum protein can be derived from the enzymatic hydrolysis of defibrinated bovine blood plasma by food-grade microbial proteases and aided with heat denaturation. The maximum degree of hydrolysis was 43% at an enzyme concentration of 110 LAPU/g protein after 15.5 hr. The resultant substrate consists of small peptides (molecular masses were less than 6.5 kDa and most were less than 1.04 kDa at maximum hydrolysis) and free amino acids, which including lysine, leucine, arginine, serine, and phenylalanine.

4. Hydrolyzed Soy Protein

Soy hydrolysate may be dephosphorylated, deglycosylated and digested by a variety of endoproteases to generate oligopeptides. The enzyme is inactivated by heat once the target molecular weight is achieved. The resultant solution may then be concentrate.

5. Hydrolyzed Collagen

As given in the CIR safety assessment and re-review of this ingredient, hydrolyzed collagen may be prepared by alkaline hydrolysis of bovine or fish collagen, followed by enzymatic hydrolysis to the desired molecular weight.

6. Hydrolyzed Elastin

Hydrolyzed elastin has been reported to be prepared from the skin of codfish or from bovine neck tendons. The fibrous tissue is washed and purified to remove soil and other residual materials and then dried. The dried elastin fibers are then hydrolyzed for several hours until the target molecular weight is reached. The final product is a solution, with the bovine source material being concentrated to a 30% active content.

7. Hydrolyzed Keratin

Hydrolyzed keratin may be prepared from sheep's wool. The wool is first washed to remove soil and debris and then boiled to remove residual oils. Next, the wool is enzyme-hydrolyzed under mild conditions for 4-6 hours. When the target molecular weight is reached, the pH is adjusted to neutralize the enzyme. The resultant solution is a mixture for hydrolyzed keratin fractions with a molecular weight of ~ 1000 Da. The solution may be diluted to produce a 30% active material.

Preservatives in Cosmetics

The majority of cosmetic preparation provides a good breeding ground for various kinds of bacterium and fungus moulds. They are almost neutral usually contain water and organic matter and often even organic nitrogen compounds and traces of mineral salts, that is provide the medium for germs growth. The consumer will reject any cosmetic product if it is contaminated with white, green, brown, or gray moulds after being opened. Chemicals with preservative properties are widely used in cosmetics to inhibit the growth of bacteria and mould. Such chemicals include halogenated phenols, hydroxyl benzoates, and formaldehyde- releasing compounds, hetrocyclic compounds such as dihydro acetic acid, alcohols, mercurials and quaternary ammonium compounds. Vitamin E is frequently used as antioxidants. The conclusion to be drawn from foregoing is simple there are hardly any cosmetics that do not require preservation for stability.

Microflora of Cosmetic Preparation

Several good reports have been published during the past few years. In some points the results of various investigators differ, which is not really surprising, since the microflora varies from product to product, even from batch to batch. The following oraganism seem to occur frequently.

Bacteria : B. Subtilis, E. coli, B. mucoides, aerobacter aerogens, pseudomonas, sarcina lutae, proteus vulgaris and *staphylococci*. All are widely spread in nature and can thrive well under the conditions prevailing at the surface of many cosmetic products.

Yeasts : Torula, manilia, and saccharomyces were identified.

Fungi : Penicillium, penicillium glaucum, rhizopus nigrideus, and recently paecilomyces were identified in cosmetic preparation.

Various preservatives are used in the cosmetic formulations such as: Bronopol, butylated hydroxytoluene (BHT), carvacrol, chlorohexidine acetate,p- Chloro-m-xylenol, 4- Chloro-3-methyl phenol, dehydroacetic acid, dichlorophene dimethoxane, fluorsalan, hexachlorophene, octyl gallate, o-phenylphenol, resorcinol, salicylanilide, zinc pyrithione, tribromsalan, benzoic acid, salicylic acid, methyl-p-hydroxy benzoate, ethyl-p-hydroxy benzoate, propyl-p-hydroxy benzoate, n-butyl-p-hydroxy benzoate, isothymol and amyl-m-cresol,

Selection of Preservatives

1. *Selection of raw materials :* Raw materials and agents that might turn the emulsion into a culture medium for fungi and bacteria are dangerous. Use sterile raw materials and an aseptic working method. Pay particular attention to the water to be used.

2. *Suitable containers and covers :* Do not use cork disk liners. If possible, sterilize or disinfect containers and covers before packing. Tubes are suitable for long storage of products.

3. Pay particular attention to O/W emulsions, especially if they contain nonionic emulsifiers.

Coloring Agents

Coloring materials in cosmetics must provide the desired tone and intensity. It is an advantage if the coloring effect is strong so that the desired result can be achieved with the smallest possible amount of dye. Tone and intensity should be as stable as possible in the preparation. The selection of coloring agents must always depend on the conditions prevailing in the preparation (pH, redox potential), fading may be caused by excessive sunlight, heat, oxidation-reduction, hydrolysis and microorganism. These considerations have let to the ever-increasing replacement of natural dyes by synthetics. A number of synthetic dyes belong to the class of materials in which some representatives are toxic, irritating or carcinogenic.

Skin compatibility not on only depends on the composition of the dyes but also on their degree of purity, and symptoms of incompatibility are often caused not by the dyes themselves but by small amounts of impurities they contain. Although it is not possible to exclude all dyes that might led to allergic reactions, since these reactions are inherently unpredictable, while some substance give rise to symptoms of allergy only very rarely indeed and others rather more frequently.

Two types of coloring agent are used in cosmetics, the soluble dyes (soluble in alcohol, water, or oil), and the insoluble pigments and lacquers; both groups can be subdivided into synthetic and natural products.

1. Natural soluble dyes

Nowadays these dyes are used comparatively rarely in cosmetics. They any be more skin compatible then synthetic dyes but their coloring power is relatively weak, their light resistance are not very good, and they are considerably more expensive in application the most widely used are alkannin, carmine, chlorophyll,henna and carotene.

2. Synthetic soluble dyes

The first synthetic dyes were synthesized from aniline; at present benzene, toluene, anthracene, and other coal-tar isolates serve as starting products for most synthetic dyes. More than thousand coal-tar dyes are known today. Only a few of them, however, can be considered for use in cosmetics. The most widely used are naphthol blue- black, indogotin, quinizarin green SS,orange I,amaranth,erythrosine J,Tartrazine and yellow AB.

3. Natural pigments

These are naturally occurring earths (aluminum silicates) whose color depends mostly on the content of hydrated iron or manganese oxides (e.g., yellow ochre, terra di Siena, red bolous, umber) these colors are completely harmless, provided they are pure. They play an important part in the coloring of powders, make-up sticks, and creams.

4. Synthetic pigments

Today, synthetic iron oxide and synthetic ochres frequently replace natural earth colors. Their hues are more intense and brighter. There is a choice of various yellow, brown-to-red, and violet shades. White synthetic pigments such as zinc oxide and titanium dioxide belong to the most important cosmetic coloring agents. Zinc oxide, in particular, not only plays a major part in decorative products but also in many other cosmetics and pharmaceutical preparations. Occasionally bismuth carbonate is also as a white pigment, while bismuth oxychloride is commonly used for pear shades.

Some cobalt compounds are used as blue synthetic pigments.

Some coal-tar dyes are also classified among the synthetic pigments; they have low solubility in water, alcohol, and oil and are therefore used in finely dispersed solid form. One of the important representatives of this group is indanthrene blue.

Many synthetic pigments (e.g., cadmium sulfide and Prussian blue) are ruled out for cosmetic preparation because of their toxicity.

5. Natural and synthetic lakes

Lakes are prepared by precipitating one or more water-soluble dyes on one or more insoluble substrates and fixing them in such a way (usually by chemical reaction) that the end product becomes a coloring agent, almost insoluble in water, oil or other solvents. Most lakes used today are prepared from synthetic dyes; an exception is "Florentine lake," which is obtained from a precipitation of carmine and brazilin (a red vegetable dye) on aluminum hydroxide. In similar manner a lake is prepared from alizarin red, a synthetic dye.

Lakes prepared from coal-tar dyes are the most important coloring agents in powders, lipsticks, and makeup. Brighter and deeper shades can be obtained with them than with pigments; they are also more colorfast than most of the soluble dyes and have good skin compatibility. When they are dry, they should be soft and friable.

The soluble dye or dyes used in the preparation of a lake determine its shade and intensity, the substrate, its covering effect. The most common substrates are zinc oxide, titanium dioxide, aluminum hydroxide, aluminum phosphate, barium phosphate, barium sulfate, magnesium carbonate, alumina hydrates and kaolin. Pigments such as zinc oxide and titanium dioxide have much higher covering power than "neutral" substances such as aluminum hydroxide. A slightly different type of lake is formed by a chemical reaction between a colorless soluble substance and an equally colorless insoluble compound, which results in an insoluble dyestuff characterized by extreme light fastness.

Herbal Excipients

Herbs or herbal ingredients are added in the form of

1. Fresh herbs/juices/pastes made from whole or part(s) of plants
2. Dried powdered herbs
3. Herbal Extracts
4. Cold expressed and/or solvent extracted, fixed oils/fats from herbs
5. Distillates/Essential Oils of herbs

4

General Instruments for Cosmetics Evaluations

General Instruments for cosmetics evaluations

With the advancements in the field of cosmetics, the involvement of different instruments have been tremendously increased in-order to obtain the scientific relevant data. Some of the instruments are enlisted below are used for this purpose:

1. Skin Surface Hydration - Corneometer® CM 825

2. Sebum on the Skin Surface - Sebumeter® SM 815

3. pH-Measurement - Skin-pH-Meter® PH 905

4. Melanin & Erythema - Mexameter® MX 18

5. Transepidermal Waterloss (TEWL) - Tewameter® TM 300

6. Skin Friction - Frictiometer® FR 700

7. Skin Temperature - Skin-Thermometer® ST 500

8. Skin Ageing - Reviscometer® RVM 600

9. Viscoelasticity by Suction - Cutometer® MPA 580

10. Measurement of the Skin Topography

11. Assessing the Skin Macro Relief by Replica & Light Transmission - Skin-Visiometer® SV 600.

12. Skin Topography directly from the Skin - Visioscan® VC 98

13. Assessing the Skin Macro Relief by Replica & Oblique Lighting - . Visioline® VL 650.

14. Special Foils for Determination of Sebum, Desquamation and other Parameters
    (a) Sebum Collector Foil - Sebufix®
    (b) Desquamation Collector Foil - Corneofix®
    (c) Skin Surface Stripping - 3S-Biokit

Corneometer

Since 1980 the Corneometer® has provided a well established method to reproducibly and accurately determine the hydration level of the skin surface. It is the world's wise used instrument for skin hydration measurement.

The Measuring Principle

The measuring principle of the Corneometer® CM 825 is based on capacitance measurement of a dielectric medium. Any change in the dielectric constant due to skin surface hydration variation alters the capacitance of a precision measuring capacitor.

Sebumeter: Determining the Skin Surface Sebum

The Sebumeter® is the most widely acknowledged, very accurate and successful sebum measurement device for skin, hair and scalp. Its use in dermatology and cosmetology is very well documented over many years with a large number of publications.

The Measuring Principle

The measurement is based on grease-spot photometry. A special tape becomes transparent in contact with the sebum on the skin surface. For sebum etermination, the measuring head of the cassette is inserted into the aperture of the device, where the transparency is measured by a light source sending light through the tape which is reflected by a little mirror behind the tape. A photocell measures the transparency. The light transmission represents the sebum content on the surface of the measuring area and is displayed in units from 0-350.

Skin-pH-Meter

The measurement of the pH-level on the skin surface is an important parameter for evaluating the quality of the hydrolipidic film on the skin especially in developing soaps, cleanser or detergents.

Mexameter: Assessing Melanin Content and Erythema Level

The human eye is very sensitive for the distinction of colours viewed side by side. But, as soon as they are seperated by space or time, differences are frequently undetected. Furthermore, the impression the eye receives from colours depends on the ambient lighting. The Mexameter® MX 18 is a very easy, quick and economical tool to measure the two components, mainly responsible for the colour of the skin: melanin and haemoglobin (erythema).

The Measuring Principle

The measurement is based on absorption/reflection. The probe of the Mexameter® MX 18 emits 3 specific light wavelengths. A receiver measures the light reflected by the skin. The positions of emitter and receiver guarantee that only diffuse and scattered light is measured. As the quantity of emitted light is defined, the quantity of light absorbed by the skin can be calculated. The melanin is measured by specific wavelengths chosen to correspond to different absorption rates by the pigments. For the erythema measurement specific wavelengths are also used, corresponding to the spectral absorption peak of haemoglobin and to avoid other colour influences (e. g., bilirubin).

Tewameter: Assessing the Skin Barrier Functions

The measurement of transepidermal waterloss (TEWL) is the most important parameter for evaluating the efficiency of the skin water barrier. Even the slightest damage in the skin water barrier can be determined at an early stage. The Tewameter® is the most accepted and best selling TEWL measurement device worldwide.

The Measuring Principle

The measurement of the water evaporation is based on the diffusion principle in an open chamber. The open chamber measurement method is the only method to assess the TEWL continuously, which are necessary for most applications without influencing the skin surface. Due to the modern, high quality electronics of the probe a stable measurement result is achieved very quickly. The probe is very easy to handle. From all TEWL measurement instruments the Tewameter® shows the most accurate values.

$$\boxed{Dm/dt = -\,D.A.\ dp/dx}$$

Where: A = surface in m^2, m = water transported (in g), t = time (h), D = diffusion constant (= 0.0877 g/m(h(mm Hg), p = vapour pressure of the atmosphere (mm Hg), x = distance from skin surface to point of measurement (m).

Skin-Thermometer: Measurement of Skin Temperature

The temperature measurement of the skin is a valuable tool for many fields of applications: besides efficacy testing and claim support for cosmetics and pharmaceuticals and objective clinical diagnosis in dermatology, there is also an application in occupational medicine, medical consultancy, and many more fields.

Reviscometer: Interesting Aspects of Skin Ageing

Determining the various parameters of the mechanical properties of skin has an established role in scientific bioengineering studies. The new aspect of the measurement - based on Resonance Running Time of the Reviscometer® RV The Reviscometer® with its unique measurement method is an ideal addition to the very well established suction measurement method of the Cutometer® and allows besides the efficacy testing of anti-ageing products, the investigation of new interesting fields such as orientation of incision during cutaneous surgery, relation between body mass index and elasticity, photoageing and many more.

Cutometer: Skin Elasticity

For many years elasticity measurements with the Cutometer® have been recognized as standard in dermatology and cosmetology and have been used to support the latest discoveries in both fields. Due to its precision and ease of use compared to other elasticity measurement methods, the Cutometer® is mentioned in most studies on this subject worldwide.

The Measuring Principle

The measuring principle is based on the suction method. Negative pressure is created in the device and the skin is drawn into the aperture of the probe. Inside the probe, the penetration depth is determined by a non-contact optical measuring system. This optical measuring system consists of a light source and a light receptor, as well as two prisms facing each other, which project the light from transmitter to receptor. The light intensity varies due to the The resistance of the skin to be sucked up by the negative pressure (firmness) and its ability to return into its original position (elasticity) are displayed as curves at the end of each measurement.

5

Herbal Cosmetics Containing Herbal Drugs

Herbal Cosmetics Containing Natural Drugs

Herbal cosmetics are natural products derived from plants, flowers, spices, fruit extracts and minerals. Herbal cosmetics have been used since ancient times and its clinical relevance have been referred in historical records. Immense benefits have been harnessed with their continued use. Our body's response to organic substances is very effective. These herbal extracts, plant derived essential oils and tinctures have amazing protective and curative properties. The preparations out of these ingredients have several benefits as cosmetic applications. Some have nourishing or cleansing actions, some whip up the circulation, others refine the pores, while some freshen the skin, leaving it soft and glowing. Many of these help skin's capacity to absorb, allowing better penetration of beneficial herbal products.

The advancements in the field of herbal ingredients and their effective approach to deliver them in an appropriate and therapeutic way has shifted the interest of consumers towards the herbal formulations. In our country, the herbal formulations have been used for centuries. The Ayurvedic system in India has a unique history spanning over 5000 years. In other countries, the popularity of herbal products has begun to rise steadily in view of increasingly visible harmful side effects of synthetic and chemical ingredients. Annual sale of herbal medications and cosmetic products in US had therefore exceeded billion just a few years ago.

Prominent Herbs used in Cosmetic Products

Some prominent herbs used for the purpose of skin rejuvenations are: Turmeric, Clove, Honey, Lemon, Amla (Indian gooseberry), Gram Flour, Henna, Lemongrass, Clove, Comfrey, Camphor, Arnica, Rose, Marigold, Sandalwood, Seaweeds and many more. These herbs are antiseptic and germicidal agents, and also exert smoothing effect on skin. These have powerful cleansing effects without any harmful side effects, and contain highly beneficial nourishing agents.

There is a large variety to choose from and modern method has enabled manufacturers to present them in ready to use bottle form with long shelf life. Some of these are natural preservatives themselves while others are hardening agents which have excellent uses for face masks. Many are excellent emulsifiers. Besides, fruits, vegetables and other herbal extracts and oils have their own fine aromas and fragrances.

Many herbs contain emollient substances, keeping the skin texture soft and smooth. Others provide rich nourishment. Chamomile is an emollient plant. Cabbage, carrot, almond, date, apricot, etc. have effective nourishing ingredients. With high vitamin and mineral contents, these rejuvenate the skin, improve skin tone and elasticity and minimize wrinkling.

Herbal products are not only good moisturizers in themselves and also act as humectants sometimes i.e., they restore moisture loss. Plant products have natural enzymes which help cleanse the skin of dead cells. Extracts of rose is in our skin toners for oily skins. It removes impurities while refining the texture and improving skin tone. Natural cleansers like milk and lemon are effective cosmetics in themselves. Fruits and vegetables such as cucumbers, peaches and apricots also make excellent face packs.

Benefits to Skin

Turmeric provides very effective germicidal treatment and skin softening remedy. It is still a part of traditional Indian beauty care in preparation for weddings. Clove is strong anti-septic agent. Honey is a strong natural moisturizer; ideal for porcelaining the skin, closing the pores and discouraging facial hair. Thyme has antiseptic properties and is effective in acne treatments. Rose water is astringent and used for closing the pores and toning the skin; its regular use slows down the aging process of the skin. Lemongrass is known for therapeutic effects; Lavender and Jasmine have essential use in aroma therapy; Amla, the Indian gooseberry, has hair-darkening properties and is among essential ingredients of many herbal hair oils. Henna has been in use internationally for centuries for hair treatment. Vegetables and Fruits are natural storehouse of beauty aids. Apricot has excellent rejuvenating effect. Papayas contain enzymes and help soften dead skin cells and remove them. Potatoes contain skin-cleaning agents. Cucumber juice benefits the area round the eyes, especially the dark circles. Lemon is a concentrate of vitamin C, increases body resistance to infection and for beauty aid can be used: as a bleach for elbows, heels and toes, as a hand lotion, as a hair rinse to make hair shining. Fuller's earth used as a pack, tightens the skin on the face and body. Sandalwood has antiseptic and germicidal effects.

The oils obtained from almond and coconut act as very good massage oils for skin and hair. The application of these oils brings a healthy glow to the skin and hair and makes them beautiful. They also help restore or maintain youth by controlling wrinkle and crease formation on the surface of the skin. Aloe Vera has well known moisturizing and nourishing properties, hence it is used commonly in herbal and organic creams, lotions and face packs.

Preparation of Herbal Cosmetics

There is a close resemblance of the method of preparation of herbal cosmetics with the conventional ones. In preparation, suitable bioactive ingredients or their extracts are used along with requisite ingredients basically used for cosmetics. It requires selection of suitable emulsifying agent, appropriate ingredient composition and modified methodology to obtain desirable product of specified parameters. Herbal cosmetics are the preparations, which represent cosmetics associated with active bioactive ingredients or pharmaceuticals. The use of phytochemicals from a variety of botanicals have double benefits like:

(i)   They are more safer than conventional cosmetics and serve for the care of whole body parts

(ii) The botanical ingredients present influence biological functions of skin and provide nutrients necessary for the healthy skin or hair.

(iii) They have in general antioxidant and skin rejuvenation effect.

In general, botanicals provide different vitamins, antioxidants, various oils, essential oils, dyes, tannins, alkaloids, carbohydrates, proteins, terpenoids and other bioactive molecules.

These are also topically applied and considered more preferred with compare to cosmetics. Personal care industry is now more concentrated on herbal based cosmetics as it is a fast growing segment with a vast scope of manifold expansion in coming years. Herbal cosmetics are not considered under the preview of Drugs and Regulations of Food and Drug Administrations. Like cosmetics, these are subjected for their safety according to the existing rules of the different countries. Generally, it is not mandatory for a manufacturer to claim that how bioactive ingredients penetrate the skin or that these ingredients cause drug-like or therapeutic effect. Some of the herbal preparations meant for skin are discussed below.

Aloe Vera Face Cleansing Lotion Formula 1

Aloe Vera Extract	2 gm
Liquid paraffin	8.8 ml
Sulfosuccinate	30 gm
Glycol Stearate	4 gm
Phenoxyethanol	1 gm
Perfume	0.2 ml
Distilled water	54 ml

General Procedure: Sulfosuccinate was taken in glass beaker and heated in 70°C. Add glycol Stearate in it and melt in same temperature with stirring. Then above solid phase I was cool for sometimes. Then liquid phase II were pouring in phase I slowly with continuous stirring. Then prepared lotion was packed and store in dark cool place.

Herbal Cleansing Cream Formula 2

Bees wax	2.0 gm
Lanolin	0.5 gm
Coconut oil	30.0 gm
Jojoba oil	20.0 gm
Borax	2.0 gm
Distilled water	35.5 gm
Preservative	q.s
Perfume	q.s

Herbal Cleansing Cream Formula 3

Bees wax	2.0 gm
Lanolin	0.5 gm
Coconut oil	20.0 gm
Jojoba oil	10.0 gm
Almond oil	20.0 gm
Borax	2.0 gm
Distilled water	35.5 gm
Preservative	q.s
Perfume	q.s

Herbal Cleansing Cream Formula 4

Bees wax	2.0 gm
Lanolin	0.5 gm
Coconut oil	20.0 gm
Wheat germ oil	30.0 gm
Borax	2.0 gm
Distilled water	35.5 gm
Preservative	q.s
Perfume	q.s

Uses

1. It can be used to moisten and nourish the skin.
2. Restore Skin pH.
3. Maintain skin vitality.

Herbal Lotion Formula 5

Myrcia oil	8 ml
Orange oil	0.5 ml
Pimenta oil	0.5 ml
Ethyl Alcohol	610.0 ml
Water	up to 1000 ml

Method: Mix the oils with the alcohol and gradually add water until the product measures 1000 ml. Set the mixture aside in well-closed container for 8 days, then filter, using 10 gm of talc, if necessary, to render the product clear.

Uses

1. It can be used to moisten and nourish the skin.
2. Also as after shave lotion.

Herbal Preparations for Hairs Formula 6

Henna Hair Dye

Formula	w/w
Henna powder	50 gm
Glycerine	5 gm
Cyclo dimethicone	4 gm
Citric acid	0.4 gm
Distilled water	40.6 ml

Method: Add the henna powder into a glass beaker, add slowly the distilled water and stir until it becomes a creamy thick paste. Then add the glycerine and stir. Then add cyclo dimethicone and stirring well. The pH should be between 3-5, test pH with pH indicator strips. If pH is above 5 you can lower with citric acid. Then formulation was pack and labelled it.

Uses

1. It can be used to nourish the hairs.
2. Natural hair colourant.
3. Proves beneficial in dry hair conditions.
4. Causes less hair fall.

Herbal Pack Formula 7

Quillaja bark powder	5%
Ammonium carbonate	1%
Borax	1%
Bay leaf oil	0.1%
Water	92%

Method: Disperse quillaja bark powder in water and then add aqueous solution of borax and ammonium carbonate slowly with stirring for few hours. Add bay leaf oil and this mixture is set-aside for few days. Then filter and pack the filtrate in to jars or bottles.

Uses

1. It can be used to moisten and nourish the hair.
2. Also as conditioner.

Herbal Anti-Ageing Preparations

Ageing is a fundamental process of life and the skin is the most visible organ making us aware of the ageing process every time. An increase in the scientific interest in reducing the appearance of ageing has lead to thrive the search of effective anti-ageing agent more prominently. As we age, the skin's pH becomes more and more neutral. The reduced acidity kills fewer bacteria, leaving the skin susceptible to bacterial growth and infections. The skin weakens as a result and begins developing problems. The aging process of the skin causes biochemical changes in collagen and elastin, the connective tissues underlying the skin, which give the skin its firmness (collagen) and elasticity (elastin). As the skin becomes less elastic, the underlying fatty tissue begins to disappear resulting in the skin beginning to sag. Our skin is less supple, and wrinkles begin to form. At this stage, our skin is more easily injured, heals more slowly and tends to dry out more quickly.

The accumulation of dermatological changes in the human skin is termed as "Skin aging". Basically there are two distinct types of aging. Aging caused by the genes is called *intrinsic* (internal) *aging*. The other type of aging is known as *extrinsic* (external) *aging* and is caused by environmental factors, such as exposure to the sun's rays. The most evident and reproducible biological feature of ageing skin is the flattening of the dermal-epidermal junction. There is a general atrophy of the extracellular matrix which is reflected by a decrease in the number of fibroblasts, reduced levels of collagen and elastin, and their organization is impaired.

Anti-Aging Agents

There are various active ingredients known to have regenerating effects in skin cells helping to slow down degenerative processes as they occur in the aging skin. Regenerative processes may include stimulation of the production of proteins (e.g., collagen, elastin), prevention of water loss, stimulation of the skin's blood circulation, replenishing the subepidermis with natural lipids, and maintenance of the natural homeostasis of the skin cell. Antioxidants like, for example, vitamin C and vitamin E are usually also used in anti-aging cosmetic products.

These are those cosmaceutical preparations which fight against the different signs of aging. Modern anti-aging preparations feature a large variety of active ingredients against skin aging.

Most of these ingredients are based on recent findings that in aging the balance between collagen synthesis and collagen fragmentation is altered. Hence, the major targets of anti-aging agents are oxidative stress and collagen metabolism. In addition, as it is known that a well-moisturized skin is less prone to oxidative injuries and premature aging, moisturizing agents form another important part of anti-aging agents.

Over 60 botanicals are marketed in cosmaceutical formulations. The most important botanicals pertaining to cosmaceutical use include teas, soy, pomegranate, date, grape seed, pycnogenol, horse chestnut, German chamomile, curcumin, comfrey, allantoin, and aloe. All are documented to treat dermatologic conditions. There is even a larger number of synthetic compounds that have been shown to have anti-aging properties. Many compounds have antioxidant functions or alter the collagen metabolism. Certain preparations which can heal and rejuvenate the signs of ageing are enlisted below.

Anti-ageing Cream Formula 1

Formula	w/w (for 100 gm)
Hyaluronic acid	2 gm
Triglyceride	12 gm

Benzyl alcohol	4 gm
Jojoba oil	9 gm
Tamarind	0.5 gm
Stearic acid	1.5 gm
Polysorbate 60	2.5 gm
EDTA	0.50 gm
Distilled water	68 ml

Anti-ageing Cream Formula 2

Formula	w/w (for 100 gm)
Hyaluronic acid	2 gm
Triglyceride	12 gm
Benzyl alcohol	4 gm
Jojoba oil	9 gm
Genistein	0.5 gm
Stearic acid	1.5 gm
Polysorbate 60	2.5 gm
EDTA	0.50 gm
Distilled water	68 ml

Anti-ageing Cream Formula 3

Wool alcohols	5 gm
Hard paraffin	25 gm
White soft paraffin	15 gm
Liquid paraffin	35.0 gm
Grape seed extract	20.0 gm
Perfume	q.s

General Method: Melt all the above ingredients except the extract and perfume. When all ingredients melt, continuously stir them and add extract slightly till it cools to 35°C. Perfume must be added at the last.

Uses

1. It prevents wrinkle formation in the skin.
2. Causes skin tightening.
3. Gives a younger look.

4. Maintain skin rejuvenation property.

5. Helpful in prevention of blemishes, dark spots etc.

Antioxidants

Antioxidants inhibit the production of Reactive Oxygen Species (ROS) by direct scavenging, decrease the amount of oxidants in and around our cells, prevent ROS from reaching their biological targets, limit the propagation of oxidants such as the one that occurs during lipid peroxidation, and thwart oxidative stress thereby preventing the aging phenomenon.

Types of Antioxidants

1. **Endogenous Antioxidants:** Endogenous antioxidants are essentially enzymes that catalytically remove oxidants. Major endogenous antioxidants are superoxide dismutase, superoxide reductase, catalase, and glutathione peroxidase. These enzymes play a key role in decreasing the content of oxidants and preventing oxidative damage. Other endogenous antioxidant molecules, such as heme oxygenase, minimize the availability of oxidants.

2. **Exogenous Antioxidants:** Exogenous antioxidants include antioxidants that cannot be synthesized by our body such as vitamins, trace elements, and phyto antioxidants. Vitamin E (tocopherol) is the most powerful liposoluble antioxidant. It inhibits the peroxidation of membrane lipids. It reacts with free radicals to form the radical tocopheryl, a stable substance that stops the chain reaction of the membrane lipids.

3. **Food-Derived Antioxidants:** Diets rich in a variety of phytoantioxidants (fruits, grains, and vegetables) are protective against several human diseases; hence the nutritional worldwide program: eat five servings of fruits and vegetables every day.

4. **Natural Antioxidants:** Plants suffer from oxidative stress induced by UV radiation as much as animals and humans do, but cannot protect themselves as humans do by exogenous means and have therefore developed multiple strategies and highly effective molecules to defend themselves against environmental stress.

Plants contain multiple antioxidants effective in ideal combinations, the so-called phyto antioxidants, capable of both protecting their own cells and extracellular matrix against oxidative stress induced by UV radiation and of conferring protection to other organisms upon ingestion or topical application.

Most phyto antioxidants belong either to polyphenols or terpenes and form a family of multiple factors from multiple plants. Polyphenols are synthesized by plants, participate in their metabolism, and contribute to their defense against environmental stresses. Polyphenols are found in roots, stems, flowers, and leaves of all plants. They differ among themselves by molecular weight, polarity, and solubility. Polyphenols contain an —OH group attached to a benzene ring.

Antioxidant is "an organic compound added to natural fats and oils and food products, to retard oxidation, deterioration, and rancidity". Many antioxidants are substituted phenolic compounds (butylated hyroxyanisole, di-tert-butyl-para-cresol and propyl gallate). Maximum concentration of antioxidants approved by FDA (Food and Drug Administration) is 0.02%-0.05%.

Choice of Antioxidants in Cosmetic Formulas

An antioxidant should possess certain physical and physiological properties if it is to be of practical value in cosmetic, pharmaceutical and food preparation:

1. The antioxidant should not impart odour or taste to the preparation to which it is added;

2. It should be nearly neutral in reaction

3. It should be easily and definitely soluble in the substrate

4. It must be pharmacologically safe and must not be strongly toxic to animal tissues.

Antioxidant preservatives are able to inhibit reactions promoted by oxygen, thus avoiding the oxidation and rancidity of commonly used fats, oils, waxes, surfactants, perfumes, antioxidants, which contain a phenolic group, play an important role in cosmetics, pharmaceutical products and food. Antioxidants further classified as natural antioxidants, are mainly represented by tocopherols, and synthetic antioxidants, like 2,6- di-tert-butyl-p-hydroxy toluene (BHT), tert-butyl-4-hydroxy anisole (BHA), propyl, octyl and dodecyl gallate, tert- butylhydroquinone (TBHQ) and nordihydroguaiaretic acid (NDGA). Some of the synthetic antioxidants used in cosmetic formulas, such as butylated hydroxyanisole (BHA) and butylated hydroxytoluene (BHT) are carcinogenic so that extensive use of such raw materials in cosmetics may represent a potential health risk. 3-tert-butyl-4-hydroxy anisole (BHA) is one of the widely used synthetic antioxidant in cosmetic preparations. This substance is generally recognized as safe for use in products, when the total content of antioxidants is not over 0.02% of fat or oil content, including essential (volatile) content of the product.

Antioxidant Cream Formula 1

Formula	(w/w) (for 25 gm)
Sesame oil	6 ml
Tamarind extract	1 gm
Lanoline	1 gm
Glycerine	2 ml
Curcumin extract	1.5 gm
EDTA	0.3 ml
Perfume	0.2 ml
Purified water	14 ml

General Procedure: Weigh 1 gm of tamarind and melt in china dish for temperature maintain in 70°C. Add curcumin and lanoline in same temperature in continuous stirring. Then phase II, liquid component sesame oil, glycerine, EDTA and water were pouring in phase I above solution in maintain stirring and temperature 40°C and then added of remaining water. After that perfume were added in final product. Packed in suitable container.

Antioxidant Cream Formula 2

Formula	(w/w) (for 25 gm)
Sesame oil	6 ml
Glycorriza extract	1 gm
Lanoline	1 gm
Glycerine	2 ml
Cinnamon extract	1.5 gm
EDTA	0.3 ml
Perfume	0.2 ml
Purified water	14 ml

Antioxidant Cream Formula 3

Formula	(w/w) (for 25 gm)
Sesame oil	6 ml
Grape Seed Extract	2 gm

Glycerine	2 ml
Aloe gel	1.5 gm
EDTA	0.3 ml
Perfume	0.2 ml
Purified water	14 ml

Antioxidant Cream Formula 4

Formula	(w/w) (for 25 gm)
Linseed oil	6 ml
Curcummin extract	1 gm
Lanoline	1 gm
Glycerine	2 ml
Ginseng extract	1.5 gm
EDTA	0.3 ml
Perfume	0.2 ml
Purified water	14 ml

Antioxidant Cream Formula 5

Formula	(w/w) (for 25 gm)
Almond oil	6 ml
Rhubarb extract	1 gm
Lanoline	1 gm
Glycerine	2 ml
Curcummber extract	1.5 gm
EDTA	0.3 ml
Perfume	0.2 ml
Rose water	14 ml

Uses

1. It helps in maintaining the elasticity of the skin.
2. Protection against reactive oxygen species generated effects.
3. Maintains cellular vitality.
4. Makes skin glow and looks younger.

Herbal Skin Toners and Tonics

A skin toner is a liquid or light lotion that is used in several different applications of skin care. Of these, the most common is to use a toner, usually with witch hazel or alcohol, to clean the skin and perhaps reduce oil and prevent acne breakouts. These are often called astringents.

Another type of toner used is called a tonic. This type typically contains a smaller amount of alcohol than do astringents, but it may still have that somewhat prickly or stingy feel that users often note when they place alcohol on the face. They also often feel cooler than plain water. Tonics do help clean the skin, and women or men who have combination type skin, with dry skin on the cheeks and more oily skin on the forehead and nose (called the T-zone), may prefer a tonic to an astringent.

The common method for applying skin toner is to dab some on a cotton ball and apply it to the face. A few toners come in spray bottles, and users just spritz the face with them. In most cases, the user doesn't have to wash off the toner, as it's meant to be a finishing step in a skin cleaning regimen. People should be careful when applying toner, especially any types that contain alcohol, and avoid getting it too close to the eyes. Individuals who have areas of the skin that are badly broken out may want to dab those areas last, so they don't transfer bacteria from one part of the skin to the other, which may result in more break. For example, a toner for oily skin will contain active substances that regulate the function of sebaceous glands, antibacterial substances, keratolytic substances that slightly peel the cells of the top layer of the skin preventing them from accumulating and blocking the pores. A toner for oily skin will definitely also contain alcohol, which removes excessive fats from the skin. A toner for normal, combined skin will contain ingredients that balance the function of sebaceous glands harmonizing the oily and dry zones of the face and refresh the skin. A toner for dry skin must contain substances that soften the skin and reduce irritation and an astringent feeling after washing.

Toner's primary job is to restore skin's natural pH balance. The pH scale is measured from 0 to 14. 7 is being neutral. The optimum pH level for skin is a slightly acidic 5.5, but varies with age. The aim for a pH of between 4.5 - 6.0 to achieve a healthy skin mantle each time after cleaning the face to restore the natural balance of acidity.

Most cleansers have a pH value between 6.5 and 8.0, which can help minimize the oil on your skin, but also rob the skin of moisture. After cleansing, your skin's pH balance becomes too high and your skin has to *work overtime* to restore the balance. By using the skin toner, the skin's pH level is immediately restored to its optimum range providing the perfect condition for serums and moisturizers to resist and fight bacteria. Some of the toners of herbal origin are discussed below.

Skin Toner Formula 1

Formula	% (w/w) (for 100 gm)
Sulfosuccinate	25 gm
Glycol stearate	5 gm
PEG-150 distearate	2.5 gm
Phenoxyethanol	2 gm
Perfume	0.4 ml
Warm distilled water	60 ml

General Procedure: First, geographically mixing of different individual compounds and keep sulfosuccinate and glycol stearate in glass beaker then heated 70°C. Add PEG-150 distearate in this mixer and melt it. Then stir melted distreate and water in phase I solution gently. Then packed in suitable container.

Skin Tonic Formula 1

Formula	% (w/w)
Ethyl alcohol	36 ml
Borax	1 gm
Tincture of benzion	2.6 ml
Glycerine	20 ml
Perfume	0.4 ml
Water	40 ml

General Procedure: Dissolve the tincture of benzion and perfume in the alcohol. Dissolve the borax in it. Mix the glycerine with water. Then add the tincture and alcohol. Mix thoroughly and filter it. Then Packed and labelled it in suitable container.

Uses

Restore skin pH.

Prevent skin infections.

Prevent sedimentation of pollutants on the skin surface.

Herbal Sunscreens

Skin is the outermost and largest organ of the body hence it is most prone to photodamage as it is directly exposed to sun light. In recent years, the incidences of ultraviolet radiation related diseases and disorders are continuously growing. When the mammalian skin is exposed long term to ultraviolet radiation, it induces the oxidative stress by generating the reactive oxygen species. These substances further trigger the development of skin cancer in Individuals. The various other biological responses occur in the skin due to UV exposure include the development of erythema, edema, sunburn cell formation, hyperplasia, immunosuppression, DNA damage, photoaging and melanogenesis. Melanin pigmentation of the skin absorbs UV light and thus protects skin cells from the detrimental effects of UV exposure. But in certain circumstances, the amount of melanin produced is not sufficient enough to protect the skin. Hence, the protection of skin from photodamage by some other means is an urgent concern. One strategy for safeguarding the skin from UV radiation is the use of sunscreens to counteract the reactive oxygen species by blocking the UV radiation exposed on the epidermis.

The use of sunscreen is a most common practice now a days that provides protection against the adverse effects of UV radiation. Many synthetic sunscreens are available in the market but they pose possible adverse side effects. Thus, the use of botanicals as sunscreen has been gaining attention in recent times. Natural substances extracted from herbs acts as the potential photoprotective resources owing to their UV absorbing property in the UV region.

In addition, they exhibit antioxidant property antimutagenic property, anti-inflammatory property and anticarcinogenic activity. So the use of botanicals is an approach to reduce the UV generated ROS-mediated photodamage, immune-suppression and skin cancer in patients

Botanicals as photoprotectives

The use of active photoprotectives from natural origin is very beneficial in combating the deleterious effects of UV rays. The important group of compounds acts as the UV blockers include phenolic acids, flavonoids and high molecular weight polyphenols. Naturally occurring phenolic acids include hydroxycinnamic acid and hydroxybenzoic acid. High molecular weight polyphenols include condensed polymers of catechins or epicatechins and hydrolysable polymers of gallic or ellagic acids. Many flavonoids such as quercetin, luteolin and catechins are found to be better antioxidants as well as good UV blocker. The following section reviews the use of certain botanicals as sun screen against photoaging and prevention of skin cancer. Some of the cosmetic sunscreen preparations are discussed below:

Herbal Sunscreen Formula 1

Linseed oil	8 ml
Orange oil	0.5 ml

Almond oil	0.5 ml
Ethyl alcohol	610 ml
Rose water up to	1000 ml

Herbal Sunscreen Formula 2

Tragacanth	2.0 gm
Glycerine	10.0 gm
Curcummin extract	20 gm
Rose water	78.0 gm
Perfume	q.s.
Preservative	q.s.

Uses

1. Protects aginst solar radiations.
2. Store skin pH.
3. Maintain skin vitality.
4. Reduce collagen and elastin damage.

Skin Pigmentation

Skin pigmentation disorder affects the color of your skin and it appears patchy and dark. When melanin cells which are responsible for the color of our skin, gets damaged or unhealthy it affects melanin production thus causing skin pigmentation. Skin pigmentation can be of different types like under pigmentation (vitiligo), hyper pigmentation. Skin pigmentation can be caused due to various reasons like over exposure to sun, hormonal changes, genetic factors, any drug reactions or congenital factors. Acne vulgaris (condition where we have excess acne/pimples) can also cause skin pigmentation is some areas. Our skin contains cells called melanocytes which produce the pigment called melanin, responsible for the color of our skin, hair and irises. When this pigment (melanin) is over produced due to certain reasons in our body, hyper pigmentation is ensured. All of us at any age must have suffered from skin pigmentation in different forms like moles, dark spot patches, birth marks and ageing spots. Early detection and treatment of skin pigmentation can relieve you form it. Some possible causes of skin pigmentation are:

1. Over exposure to sun
2. Hormonal changes in body

3. Heredity Reaction to some medicines

4. Acne/pimples

5. Ageing

6. More pigment formation in skin

There are various herbal treatments available for the problem for pigmentation. Some of the herbs playing crucial role in combating pigmentation problems are enlisted below:

1. Licorice (*Glycyrrhiza glabra*)

2. Rhubarb (*Rheum officinale*)

3. Bearberry (*Arctostaphylos uva-ursi*)

4. Ginseng (*Panax ginseng*)

5. Aloe (*Aloe vera*)

6. Wild Yam (*Dioscorea villosa*)

7. Japana Roxa (*Eupatorium triplinerve Vahl*)

8. Oregano (*Origanum vulgare, O. majorana*)

9. Pineaple (*Ananas comosus*)

10. Evening primrose (*Oenothera biennis*)

11. Persimmon (*Diospyros kaki*)

12. Rosehips (*Rosa canina*)

13. Ginger (*Zingiber officinale*)

14. Raspberry (*Rubus idaeus*)

15. Mulberry (*Morus alba*)

Some of the herbal formulations effective against skin pigmentation are discussed below:

Formula 1

Almond oil	5.0 gm
Glycerine	5.0 gm
Aloe gel	25.0 gm
Cucummber extract	15 gm
Rose water	50.0 gm
Preservative	q.s.

Formula 2

Paraffin wax	26.0 gm
Liquorice extract	10.0 gm
Grape seed extract	10.0 gm
Petrolium Jelly	54.0 gm
Perfume	q.s.

Uses

1. Protects against harmful radiations of the sun.
2. Protects from darkening of the skin.
3. Decrease pigmentation.
4. Prevents formation of dark spots, blemishes, pits on the skin.

6

Essentials of Stability Testing of Cosmetics

Essentials of Stability Testing of Cosmetics

Stability studies on cosmetic products supply information that indicates the relative stability level of a product under the various conditions that it can be subjected to from the moment it is manufactured until the end of its validity. This stability is relative as it varies with time and in response factors that accelerate or retard alterations in the parameters of the product. Modification within established limits do not necessarily constitute a reason for withdrawing approval of the product.

The study of cosmetic products stability contributes towards:

1. Guiding the development of the formulation and of adequate containing materials.

2. Supplying subsidies for formulation improvement.

3. Estimating the validity term and supplying information to confirm it.

Assisting in the monitoring of organoleptic, physical, chemical and microbiological stability, by producing information about the trustworthiness and safety of products.

The purpose of stability testing cosmetic products is to ensure that a new or modified product meets the intended physical, chemical and microbiological quality standards as well as functionality and aesthetics when stored under appropriate conditions.

The parameters to be evaluated must be defined by the formulator and depend on the characteristics of the product that is being studied and on the ingredients being used in the formulation. Generally they are:

Organoleptic Parameters

1. Appearance
2. Color
3. Odor and Flavour

Physical and Chemical Parameters

1. pH Value
2. Viscosity
3. Density

Microbiological Parameters

Microbial count and challenge test of the preserving system made before and/or after the accelerated study period.

A reference sample must also be taken, also known as a standard sample, which generally can be kept in the refrigerator or at room temperature, protected from light. In a complementary manner, samples from the market of products with a known acceptability or of other similar products deemed to be satisfactory in relation to the parameters being evaluated, may be used as standards.

Because of the wide variety of cosmetic products "standard" stability tests cannot be prescribed. Manufacturers require the flexibility to modify testing protocols and to build a sound scientific basis for assessing stability of their own products. Thus, specific tests may be developed in order to address new or unusual technologies, or to be adapted to products having extended shelf lives.

In general, stability tests can be conducted in real time or under accelerated conditions and should address the stability of a product under appropriate conditions of storage, transport and use.

1. Physical/Chemical Stability Tests

These describe approaches to predicting how well cosmetics will resist common stresses such as temperature extremes and light. Typically, manufacturers determine whether to perform such specialized testing based on the vulnerabilities of the particular cosmetic product and its anticipated shipping, storage display and use conditions.

Common Test Procedures

Temperature variations: High temperature testing is now commonly used as a predictor of long-term stability. Most companies conduct their high temperature testing at 37°C (98°F) and 45°C (113°F). If a product is stored at 45°C for three months (and exhibits acceptable stability) then it should be stable at room temperature for two years. Of course, the product must be stored at 25°C (77°F) for a period of one year. A good control temperature is 4°C (39°F) where most products will exhibit excellent stability. The product should also be subjected to -10°C (14°F) for three months.

Cycle testing: The product should pass three cycles of temperature testing from -10°C (14°F) to 25°C (77°F). Place the product at 10°C for 24 hours and place it at room temperature (25°C) for 24 hours. This completes one cycle. If the product passes three cycles then you can have a good degree of confidence in the stability of the product. An even more rigorous test is a -10°C to 45°C five-cycle test. This puts emulsions under a tremendous stress and, if it passes the test, indicates that you have a really stable product.

Centrifuge testing: The dispersed phase (of an oil-in-water emulsion) has a tendency to separate and rise to the top of the emulsion forming a layer of oil droplets. This phenomenon is called creaming. Creaming is one of the first signs of impending emulsion instability and should be taken seriously. A good test method to predict creaming is centrifugation. Heat the emulsion to 50°C (122°F) and centrifuge it for thirty minutes at 3000 rpm. Then inspect the resultant product for signs of creaming. This test is an absolute necessity for those products that contain powders of any kind such as liquid/cream make-up.

Light testing: Both formulas and packaging can be sensitive to the UV radiation. All products should be placed, in glass and the actual package, in the window and if its available a light box that has a broad-spectrum output. Place another glass jar completely covered with aluminum foil in the window to serve as a control. All too often we will see significant discoloration of the product and sometimes of the package also. This discoloration may be due to the fragrance or some other sensitive ingredient. Usually all that is needed is the addition of a UV absorber (e.g., 0.1% of benzophenone).

Mechanical shock testing: In order to determine whether or not shipping movements may damage the cosmetic and its packaging mechanical shock testing is often conducted. Vibration testing (e.g., on a pallet shaker) can help to determine whether de-mixing (separation) of powders or granular products is likely to occur.

Parameters to monitor: For all the above mentioned tests you should monitor the color, odor/fragrance, viscosity, pH value, and, if available, particle size uniformity and/or particle agglomeration under the microscope.

2. Microbiological Stability Tests

Microbial contaminants usually come from two different origins: during production and filling, and during the use of the cosmetic by the consumer. From the moment the cosmetic unit is opened by the consumer, a permanent microbial contamination of the cosmetic is introduced caused by contact with the consumer's hands and body. Mmicrobial preservation of cosmetics is important to ensure the microbial safety of cosmetics for the consumer, maintain the quality of the product, and confirm hygienic and high-quality handling. Although only a small number of cases of microbial infections of the consumer has been reported, microbial contamination of cosmetic products may spoil them or seriously reduce the intended quality.

Therefore, it is necessary to carry out routine microbiological analysis of each batch of the finished product coming on the market. *Pseudomonas aeruginosa, Staphylococcus aureus* and *Candida albicans* are considered the main potential pathogens in cosmetic products. These specific potential pathogens must not be detectable in 0.1 gm or 0.1 ml of a cosmetic product. The parameters examined, the criteria and methods used, and the results obtained per batch should be documented.

Common Test Procedures

Screening tests: There are various easy testing kits available on the market (e.g., dip-slides or plate counts) which provide quick and semi-quantitative results whether a cosmetic product is significantly contaminated or not. Sampling and evaluation of the results is simple and can be performed also by personnel without any microbiological training.

Quantitative tests: Quantitative tests determine the actual count level of bacteria, mold and yeast in a cosmetic product. These tests are very sophisticated and laborious and can be performed only by professional microbiological testing laboratories. Typically, methods for isolation of microorganisms from cosmetic products include direct colony counts and enrichment culturing.

3. Packaging Stability Tests

Packaging can directly affect finished product stability because of interactions which can occur between the product, the package, and the external environment. For example, product constituents may be absorbed into the container or may chemically react with the container. In addition, the container may not fully protect the product from the adverse effects of atmospheric oxygen and/or water vapor, or volatile product constituents (e.g., fragrances) may evaporate through the container.

Common Test Procedures

Glass tests: Glass is the most inert material and does not react with a cosmetic product in any way. For this reason all testing should be done in glass and the actual packaging. In this way you can determine if the cause of product failure is the formula or the package.

Weight loss tests: To determine evaporation (water loss through the container wall or closure gaps) weight loss evaluation is one of the most important tests that must be conducted. This testing (performed in the actual package with the cap torque to 100% of target torque) is done at room temperature and at 45°C (113°F) for a period of three months. The weight loss should not exceed 1% per month for the package to be considered acceptable.

Leaking tests: It may be advisable to test the packaged product in various orientations (upright, inverted, on its side, etc.) to determine whether the packaging may leak (especially during transport).

4. Test of compatibility between formulation and containing material

The stability of the product and its compatibility with the containing material are distinct concepts, separate and complementary, that must be applied to the product before it is commercialized. In this test, several alternative containing materials are analyzed to determine which is most suitable for the product.

Cellulose Packaging

Examples: Cartridges, trays, displays and cardboard packages.

Evaluated For:

1. Alterations in the paper and formulation structure, checking for possible migration of components that could contaminate the product (e.g.: sachets).
2. Physical-chemical stability of the packaging.
3. Alterations in the formulation – appearance, color, odor, among others.
4. Appearance and functionality of the package.

5. Barrier function (e.g., permeation of oil, water or gases).

6. Metal determination, whenever applicable.

Metal Packaging

Evaluated For:

1. Delamination, when applicable.

2. Corrosion.

3. Alterations in the formulation – appearance, color, odor, among others.

4. Appearance and functionality of the package.

5. Formula reaction.

6. Polish or resin integrity (internal and external).

7. Metal determination, whenever applicable.

8. Functionality.

Plastic packaging

Types of plastic: Polypropylene (PP), high density Polyethylene (HDPE), low density Polyethylene (LDPE), Polyethylene Terephthalate (PET), Polystyrene (PS) and Poly vinyl chloride (PVC).

Evaluated For:

1. Alterations in the formulation – appearance, color, odor, among others.

2. Appearance and functionality of the package.

3. Interaction and migration of components between package and product.

4. Porosity to water vapour.

5. Light transmission.

6. Heat-sealing (whenever applicable).

7. Deformity (collapse or bending).

Glass packaging

Evaluated For:

1. Alterations in the formulations – appearance, color, odor, among others.

2. Appearance and functionality of the package.

3. Mechanical resistance of the package.

Pressurized packaging

The evaluations must be in conformity with the characteristics of the previously related materials and also consider the influence of the propellant on the formulation and on the package materials.

Evaluated For:

1. Performance of the product in accordance with its functionality.
2. Corrosion and electrolysis of the package.
3. Internal and external polish control (porosity), whenever applicable.
4. Homogeneity of coatings and linings - bubble formation, fissures and corrosion.
5. Performance of the valve and it's components.
6. Presence of electrolytes, odor and formulation precipitation.

7

Assessment of Toxicity of Cosmaceuticals

Assessment of Toxicity of Cosmaceuticals

The assessment of the toxicological effects of the substances is the first step in the safety assessment. The safety assessment must be based on data on the substances and the test results regarding the properties mentioned below. There may be instances when it does not appear to be necessary or to be technically possible to provide the information: In such cases scientific justification needs to be given. Toxicological profile can be studied in terms of:

1. Acute toxicity
2. Irritation and dermal corrosiveness
    (a) Skin irritation and skin corrosiveness
    (b) Mucous membrane irritation
3. Skin sensitization
4. Dermal/percutaneous absorption
5. Repeated dose toxicity
6. Mutagenicity/genotoxicity
7. Carcinogenicity
8. Reproductive toxicity
9. Toxicokinetic studies
10. Photo-induced toxicity
    (a) Phototoxicity (photoirritation) and photosensitization
    (b) Photomutagenicity/Photoclastogenicity

1. Acute Toxicity

It is evaluated to describe the adverse effects on health, which may result from a single exposure to a substance *via* the oral, dermal or inhalation route. The *in vivo* acute oral toxicity test was originally developed to determine the LD_{50}-value (the dose at which 50% of the animal die) of the compound under investigation. It has recently been replaced by alternative methods that include the fixed dose method, acute toxic class method and the up-and-down procedure.

2. Irritation and Dermal Corrosiveness

This is evaluated in terms of skin irritation, skin corrosiveness and mucous membrane irritation produced by cosmetic ingredients.

(a) Skin Irritation and Skin Corrosiveness

Skin irritation tests have been developed to assess the potential of a certain substance to cause redness and edema after a single topical application and skin corrosion tests assess the potential of a substance to cause irreversible necrosis through the epidermis and into the dermis, following the application of a test substance for a duration length of 3 minutes up to 4 hours. Corrosive reactions are notified by formation of ulcers, bleeding, and scabs. At the end 14 days, discoloration of the skin, alopecia, and scars will be observed to assess the extent of skin corrosion reactions.

(b) Mucous Membrane Irritation

Mucous membrane irritation is accessed by determining ocular irritation produced by cosmetic ingredients after a single application. Ocular irritation tests have been developed to assess the potential of a certain substance to cause chemosis, discharge, redness to the conjunctiva, swelling of the iris and opacity to the cornea. Classical *in vivo* ocular irritation tests and the HET-CAM (Hen's Egg Test - Chorio Allantoic Membrane) test is a valid *in vitro* alternative method for evaluating mucous membrane irritation.

3. Skin Sensitization

A skin sensitizer is an agent that is able to cause an allergic response in susceptible individuals. Three common *in vivo* laboratory animal test methods are widely being used to evaluate the potential of a substance to cause skin sensitization. These tests include the Local Lymph Node Assay (LLNA), Guinea Pig Maximization Test (GPMT) and Buehler test. To date there is no validated *in vitro* test method accepted for skin sensitization.

4. Dermal/Percutaneous Absorption

Human exposure to cosmetic ingredients occurs mainly *via* transdermal absorption. In order to reach the circulation cosmetic ingredients must cross a number of cell layers of the skin. Skin is mainly divided into three layer epidermis, dermis, and subcutaneous (hypodermis) layer. Epidermis is consist of five layers, starting from the outermost layer stratum corneum, stratum lucidum, stratum granulosum, stratum spinosum to basal layer stratum basale. The *in vivo* and *in vitro* dermal/percutaneous absorption studies have been described by several international bodies. Dermal/percutaneous absorption is the amount of dermally applied substance remaining in the residual skin (excluding the stratum corneum) plus the amount of dermally applied substance which has passed through the skin and is detected in the receptor fluid. The sum is considered to be systemically available.

5. Repeated Dose Toxicity

Repeated dose toxicity comprises the adverse general toxicological effects occurring as a result of repeated daily dosing with exposure to a substance for a specific part of the expected lifespan of the test species. The 28-day and 90-day oral toxicity studies in rodents are the most commonly used repeated dose toxicity tests and often give a clear indication of target organ effects and type(s) of systemic toxicity. Currently no validated or generally accepted alternative methods are available for replacing this type of animal testing.

6. Mutagenicity/Genotoxicity

Mutagenicity refers to the induction of permanent transmissible changes in the amount or structure of the genetic material of cells or organisms. Genotoxicity is a broader term and refers to potentially harmful effects on genetic material that are not necessarily associated with mutagenicity. Several *in vitro* gene mutation test and *in vivo* tests are available and have been described for evaluating mutagenicity and genotoxicity of cosmetic ingredients, but for most cosmetic ingredients, *in vivo* tests are not considered imperative. For testing the potential genotoxicity/mutagenicity/carcinogenicity potential of oxidative hair dye ingredients a new strategy was adopted by the SCCNFP in June 2003.

Under this strategy hair dye products are evaluated by performing various *in vitro* and *in vivo* assays. Bacterial Reverse Mutation Assay, Mammalian Chromosome Aberration Test, Mammalian Cell Gene Mutation Test, DNA Damage and Repair/Unscheduled Synthesis in

Mammalian Cells, Mammalian Micronucleus Test and Syrian Hamster Embryo (SHE) Cell Transformation Assay these six assays are used to carry out *in vitro* evaluation for determining mutagenicity/genotoxicity and also the nongenotoxic/carcinogenic potential of hair dye ingredients. The aim of the *in vivo* assays is to ascertain whether a genotoxic/mutagenic effect shown *in vitro* may also occur in somatic cells under *in vivo* conditions. Mammalian Erythrocyte Micronucleus Test, Mammalian Bone Marrow Chromosome Aberration Test and Unscheduled DNA Synthesis (UDS) Test with Mammalian Liver Cells are the main assays carried under the *in vivo* evaluation of hair dyes.

7. Carcinogenicity

Substances are defined as carcinogenic if they induce tumours, increase their incidence and/or malignancy when they are inhaled, ingested, dermally applied or injected. *In vivo* carcinogenicity tests and the *in vitro* Syrian Hamster Embryo Transformation Test is the most commonly performed methodologies to evaluate carcinogenic action of cosmetic ingredients.

8. Reproductive Toxicity

Reproductive toxicity is used to describe the adverse effects induced by a substance on any aspect of mammalian reproduction. The most commonly performed *in vivo* reproduction toxicity studies are those that characterize the teratogenicity potential. Three alternative *in vitro* methods Whole Embryo Culture test (WEC), Micro Mass test (MM) and Embryotoxic Stem cell Test (EST) are used to evaluate reproductive toxicity of cosmetic ingredients.

9. Toxicokinetic Studies

Toxicokinetic studies describe the time-dependent fate of a substance within the body. This includes absorption, distribution, biotransformation (metabolism) and its excretion. In specific cases, *in vivo* or *in vitro* biotransformation studies are required to prove and to exclude certain adverse effects associated with cosmetic ingredients. Several *in vitro* models (hepatocytes in suspension or culture) are suitable for biotransformation studies; however, none of these models has been validated since so far for evaluation purpose. Finally, toxicokinetic studies are of importance in extrapolating both *in vitro* and *in vivo* animal data to man (a process termed as allometric scaling).

10. Photo-Induced Toxicity

Photo-induced toxicity is measured in terms of the photoirritation and photomutagenicity potential of cosmetic ingredients.

(a) Photoirritation/Photosensitization

In vitro method for the determination of the photoxicological profile of all UV light absorbing chemicals and especially for those cosmetic ingredients to be used as UV filters.

(b) Photomutagenicity/Photogenotoxicity

Photomutagenicity/photogenotoxicity test is desirable for assessing the UV radiation absorbing potential of cosmetic ingredients as adapted by SCC, guidelines in 1990.

8

List of Cosmetics : Formulation, Method of Preparation and Uses

Exercise - 1

Object : To prepare and pack "Face Pack"

Formula :

Grain meal	:	25%
Crushed almond meal	:	10%
Talc	:	15%
Glycerol	:	25%
Water, de-ionized	:	25%
Color, perfume, preservative	:	q.s.

Method : Dry materials are blended together thoroughly, then add water slowly with stirring in which glycerol is pre added. If color and preservative are adding, it is added in dry ingredient first. Lastly add the perfume in paste and mix well.

Use : For cleaning facial skin.

Exercise - 2

Object : To prepare "Face Pack"

Formula :

Bentonite	:	15%
Titanium dioxide	:	2%
Glycerol	:	4%
Sulfonated vegetable oil	:	3%
Water	:	76%
Color, perfume, preservative	:	q.s.

Method :

(i)   Fine solid particles are pre-blended.

(ii)   Glycerol is added to water.

(iii) Add dry powder in aqueous solution with stirring.

(iii) Then add sulfonated vegetable oil very slowly with homogeneous mixing.

(iv)   Make up the volume with stirring.

Use : It produces cleaning effect by absorption and by removal of harder film after drying and also shows lightening effect.

Exercise - 3

Object : To prepare and pack "Face Mask".

Formula :

Isopropyl myristate	:	31.5%
Titanium dioxide/ or pigment/talcum	:	35.5%
Ozokerite (80 – 88% M.P.)	:	17.5%
Cetyl alcohol	:	2.5%
Sorbitan mono-oleate (or Span. 80)	:	6.5%
Polyoxyethylene sorbitan mono-oleate	:	6.5%
Perfume	:	q.s.

Method : Melt all ingredients except powder at the temperature as low as possible, and then add the finely pulverized powders. Homogenize the mass and heat to 55°C and stir slowly to remove the air. Pour it into the container and allow cooling.

Use : As pancake make-up and improving glow of face skin.

Exercise - 4

Object : To prepare and pack "Face Mask".

Formula :

A - Part :	Stearic acid	:	15.0 gm
	Span 60	:	2.5 gm
	Isopropyl palmitate	:	2.0 gm
B - Part :	Tween 60	:	1.5 gm
	Propylene glycol	:	10.0 gm
	Water	:	54.0 gm
	Dry powder (TiO2 /Talc) and Inorganic pigment	:	15.0 gm
	Perfume	:	q.s.
	Preservative	:	q.s.
	Dry powder: -talcum	:	8 gm
	TiO_2	:	2 gm
	Iron oxide lead	:	1.0 gm

Method :

1. Mix the color (Pigment) and talc to disperse the color properly.
2. Heat all components of A at 85°C.
3. Heat all components of B separately at 90°C.
4. Add B part to A part with continuous stirring and cool.
5. Add perfume when the temperature comes down to 35°C.
6. Preservative is added in water of component B before cream is made.

Use : As masking of freckles, small birthmarks, enlarged follicle mouths (or pore skin) acne, scars of skin lesions.

Exercise - 5

Object : To prepare and evaluate Cold Cream.

Formula :

Part (A)	Bees wax	:	8.0 gm
	Mineral oil	:	49.0 gm
	Paraffin wax	:	7.0 gm
	Cetyl alcohol	:	1.0 gm
Part (B)	Borax	:	0.4 gm
	Water	:	34.6 gm
	Preservative (Phenol)	:	q.s. (0.1%)
Part (C)	Perfume	:	q.s.

Method : Melt all the ingredients of part A gradually by their increasing melting point with stirring. Take separately Part B material and mix properly and heat at same temperature of Part A. Mix two phases with continuous stirring until a smooth cream is formed. Then, add perfume cool the cream properly, then fill it in a suitable container.

Evaluation :

(i)	Rheology	:	Determine its viscosity and Spreadability.
	Viscosity	:	1:10 dilution by Viscometer.
(ii)	Sensitivity	:	Tested on before hand by patch testing ($1cm^2$ on skin either open or exclusive.
	Photosensitivity	:	Apply patches on skin; keep for 15 minutes under sun – test its sensitivity.
(iii)	Quantitative estimation of ingredients.		
(iv)	Grittiness	:	Rub a pinch of cream between fingers and thumps then observe for rashes or eruptions.

Use : As an emollient.

Exercise - 6

Object : To prepare and pack "Cold Cream".

Formula :

Cetyl esters wax	:	125 gm
White wax	:	120 gm
Mineral oil	:	560 gm
Sodium borate	:	5 gm
Purified water	:	190 ml

Method : Reduce the cetyl ester wax and the white wax to small pieces, melt them on a steam bath with the mineral oil, and continue heating until the temperature of the mixture reaches at 70°C. Dissolve sodium borate in purified water and warm up to 70°C, then gradually add the warm solution to the melted mixture, stirring rapidly and continuously until it has congealed.

Use : As an emollient, cleaning cream and ointment base.

Exercise - 7

Object : To prepare and pack "Cold Cream".

Formula :

Almond oil (Sweet)	:	80%
Bees wax	:	10%
Spermaceti	:	10%

Method : Melt all ingredients with increasing melting point by continuous stirring up to cooling.

Use : As moisturizer

As covering agent for sharp edges of the corneal disks

As barrier film for foreign material penetration

As skin nutrient emollient cream

Exercise - 8

Object : To prepare and pack "Cold Cream".

Formula :

Ceratum craleni

Cera-alba (bleached bees wax)   :   12 gm

Almond oil   :   50 gm

Rose water   :   37.5 ml

Method : Firstly melt wax and oil together, then rose water is added under intensive stirring.

Use : As an emollient.

As skin nourishing cream.

Exercise - 9

Object : To prepare Cold Cream.

Formula :

Cera-alba (bleached bees wax)	:	7.0 gm
Spermaceti	:	8.0 gm
Almond oil	:	60.0 gm
Water	:	25 gm
Attar or Roses	:	2 drops

Method : Melt all the waxes and then add almond oil with continuous stirring until it cool. Then add water and finally attar or roses are added under intensive stirring.

Use : As an emollient.

Exercise - 10

Object : To prepare and pack "Vanishing Cream".

Formula :

Stearic acid	:	20 gm
Potassium hydroxide	:	1.4 gm
Glycerin	:	4.0 gm
Water	:	74.6 gm
Perfume	:	q.s.
Preservative	:	q.s.

Method : Firstly heat stearic acid and potassium hydroxide at 70°C in a crucible. Then dissolve all the ingredients in water with continuous stirring. Cool it to 35°C with stirring and then add perfume lastly.

Use : As masking cream.

Exercise - 11

Object : To prepare and pack "Vanishing Cream".

Formula :

Phase A	Bees wax	:	20%
	Mineral oil	:	45%
	Cetyl alcohol	:	2.0%
	Cholesterol	:	2.5%
	Cocoa butter	:	7.0%
	Propylparabane	:	0.15%
	Anti-oxidant	:	0.05%
Phase B	Methylparabane	:	0.15%
	Borax	:	1.0%
	Water	:	21.80%
	Perfume	:	0.35%

Method : Add phase A (at 75°C) very slowly to the phase B (at 75°C) of emulsion. Stir it continuously and homogenize to assure efficient emulsification. Cool it at 50°C and add perfumes it suitably.

Use : To hide the blemishes of skin.

Exercise - 12

Object : To prepare and pack "Vanishing Cream".

Formula :

Phase A	Glyceryl monostearate	:	10.0%
	Lanolin	:	2.0%
	Methylparabane	:	0.1%
Phase B	Glycerin	:	15.0%
	Stearyl calaminoformyl methyl	:	1.5%
	Oyridinium chloride	:	
	Purified Water q.s.	:	100%
	Perfume	:	q.s.

Method : Melt phase A then mix separately all ingredients of phase B. Mix phase A slowly to phase B at same temperature with continuous stirring. Cool at room temperature then add perfume and pack in to suitable container.

Use : As protective.

Exercise - 13

Object : To prepare and pack "Vanishing Cream".

Formula :

Phase A	Stearic acid	:	13.0%
	Stearyl alcohol	:	1.0%
	Cetyl alcohol	:	1.0%
	Methylparabane	:	0.10%
Phase B	Propylparabane	:	0.05%
	Glycerin	:	10.0%
	Potassium hydroxide	:	0.90%
	Perfumed Water q.s.	:	100%

Method : Melt Phase A ingredient with increasing order of melting point up to 70°C. Then make separate Phase B at the same temprature. Mix oil phase slowly with stirring in to the water phase till mixture cool up to room temperature. Add perfume and fill in to suitable container.

Use : As protective or mask for skin.

Exercise - 14

Object : To prepare and pack "Cleansing Cream".

Formula :

Bees wax	:	16.67%
Mineral oil	:	50%
Borax	:	0.83%
Water	:	32.50%

Method : Melt the bees wax and mineral oil together and bring a temperature at 70^0C. Dissolve borax in water and bring the temperature of this solution up to 70°C. Add water phase into oil phase with rapid stirring. After addition of water stir slowly; while cooling, add perfume at temperature 50°C. Fill in to jars when cream has cooled to 42°C.

Use : For cleansing the skin

Exercise - 15

Object : To prepare and pack "Cleansing Cream".

Formula :

Mineral oil 65/75	:	38%
Bees wax	:	3%
Spermaceti	:	3%
Glycerol	:	4%
Glyceryl monostearate	:	12%
Water	:	40%

Method : Melt together all the waxes and oil and keep the temperature up to 70ºC. Heat glycerol and water together at 70ºC, add oil phase to water phase with rapid stirring and add perfume at 50ºC. Agitate until cooled to about 45ºC then pour in to suitable container.

Use : For cleaning the skin.

Exercise - 16

Object : To prepare and pack "Cleansing Cream".

Formula :

Spermaceti	:	12.5%
Beeswax	:	12%
Expressed almond oil	:	56.0%
(or Percic Oil)		
Borax	:	0.5%
Rose water	:	5%
Distilled water	:	15%
Rose oil	:	q.s.

Method : Make oil phase by mixing melted spermaceti, bees wax and expressed almond oil and separately make water phase by dissolve borax in to distilled water in which rose water already added. Add water phase slowly with stirring in to oil phase. When thoroughly mixed, add rose oil homogeneously and pack in to tubes or jars.

Use : As cleaning agent for normal skin.

Exercise - 17

Object : To prepare and pack "Cleansing Cream".

Formula :

Mineral oil	:	35%
Spermaceti	:	8%
Glycerol	:	5%
Glycol stearate	:	10%
Paraffin	:	5%
Water	:	37%

Method : Melt together all the waxes and oil and bring the temperature up to 70°C. Heat glycerol and water together at 70°C. Add oil phase into water phase with rapid stirring. Add perfume at 50°C. Agitate until cooled to about 45°C and then pour in to jar.

Use : For cleaning as well as to prevent dryness.

Exercise - 18

Object : To prepare and pack "After Shave Lotions".

Formula :

Ethyl alcohol 95%		
especially denatured	:	80.5%
Water demineralized	:	5%
Sodium stearate	:	6%
Glycerol	:	4%
Propylene glycol	:	3%
Perfume oil	:	0.1%

Method : Place all ingredients except the perfume oil in a closed stainless steel glass lined steam jacket fitted with an agitator and a water cooled condenser. Heat with stirring and when the temperature reaches about 55°C, add the perfume oil. Continue heating and stir until completely dissolved. Adjust temperature up to 70°C to 74°C and pour in to moulds. Color if desired, is added by dissolving it in the water of the formulation.

Use : To provide soft and smooth feeling, cooling effect, astringent and disinfectant.

Exercise - 19

Object : To prepare and pack "After Shave Lotion".

Formula :

Alcohol 96%	:	32.6%
Water	:	40%
Birch extract	:	10%
Aluminum acetate	:	10%
Lactic acid 80%	:	1%
Perfume oil	:	0.5%

Method : Mix the alcoholic solution of perfume oil and aqueous solution of lactic acid. Add birch extract and aluminum acetate and filter the solution.

Use : For refreshing and healing of small cuts.

Exercise - 20

Object : To prepare and pack "After Shave Lotion".

Formula :

Oily Phase	Alcoholic acid	:	1%
	Stearic acid	:	3.0%
	Mineral oil	:	1.0%
	Propylparabane	:	0.15%
Water Phase	Methylparabane	:	0.15%
	Triethanolamine	:	1.5%
	Water	:	83.90%
	Perfume	:	0.30%

Method : Mix oily phase ingredients and water phase ingredients at 75°C separately. Add both the phases slowly with stirring. Cool the solution at 35°C and add perfume.

Use : As an emollient.

Exercise - 21

Object : To prepare and evaluate "After Shave Cream".

Formula :

Oily Phase	Lanolin	:	28.00%
	Bees wax	:	14.00%
	Vegetable oil	:	20.00%
	Mineral oil (65/75)	:	10%
	Cholesterol	:	2.0%
	Propylparabane	:	0.15%
	Anti-oxidant	:	0.05%
Water Phase	Methylparabane	:	0.15%
	Borax	:	0.80%
	Water	:	24.60%
	Perfume	:	0.25%

Method : Prepare oily phase and water phase separately. Add water phase svery slowly into oily phase (oily phase) at 75°C. Stir constantly and homogenize to ensure efficient emulsification. Cool and add with stirring perfume at 40 – 50°C.

Use : For refreshing and healing of small cuts.

Exercise - 22

Object : To prepare and pack "Acid balanced Shampoo".

Formula :

Coconut oil	:	18.0%
Castor oil	:	4.0%
Potassium hydroxide (85%)	:	5.3%
Glycerol	:	4.0%
Perfume	:	0.2%
Water	:	68%
Borax	:	0.5%

Method : Make oil and water soluble solution properly. Mix gradually oil phase in to water phases slowly. Add perfume lastly with thorough mixing and fill in to containers.

Use : For cleaning of the hair and scalp.

Exercise - 23

Object : To prepare and pack "Acid balanced Shampoo".

Formula :

Coconut oil	:	21.0%
Potassium hydroxide 85%	:	4.1%
Water	:	54%
Perfume	:	0.5%
Olive oil	:	3.0%
Sodium hydroxide 95%	:	1.9%
Ethyl alcohol	:	15%
Ethylene diamine		
Tetra acetic acid	:	0.5%

Method : Mix the oily water-soluble ingredients separately. Mix gradually oil and water phases. Add perfume lastly with stirring.

Use : For cleaning of the hair and scalp.

Exercise - 24

Object : To prepare and pack "Egg Shampoo".

Formula :

Fatty alcohol sulphate	:	27.50 gm
Lauryl isopropanilamide	:	1.0 gm
Ethylene glycol monostearate	:	3.00 gm
Egg powder	:	0.25 gm
Perfume	:	q.s.
Preservative	:	q.s.

Method : Add egg powder with small quantity of water to make a paste. Dilute it with some amount of detergent. Mix other ingredients with water separately. Add the first mixture to it with continuous stirring. Then lastly add perfume.

Use : For the conditioning along with cleaning of hairs.

Exercise - 25

Object : To prepare and pack "Egg Shampoo".

Formula :

Egg powder	:	10%
Atlas G -1441	:	1%
Alcohol 95%	:	5%
Protein fatty acid		
Condensation product (25%)	:	10%
Triethanolamine lauryl sulphate (50%)	:	40%
Water	:	34%

Method : Mix triethanolamine lauryl sulphate and protein fatty acid condensation product. Add 95% alcohol and a part of water and stir it. Make the dispersion of egg yolk in water and combine both the solutions with stirring to make cream. Add melted atlas G – 1441 (a polyoxyethylene sorbitol lanolin derivative) to the mixture with continuous stirring to homogenize it.

Use : As hair conditioner.

As protective colloid

As fat restoring agent in hairs

Exercise - 26

Object : To prepare and evaluate "Talcum Powder".

Formula :

Talc	:	75.0 gm
Colloidal kaolin	:	10.0 gm
Colloidal silica	:	5.0 gm
Magnesium carbonate	:	5.0 gm
Aluminum stearate	:	4.0 gm
Boric acid	:	0.3 gm
Perfume	:	0.7 gm

Method : Mix perfumes with magnesium carbonate and keeps it aside for some time. Mix other ingredients properly which are finely powdered previously. Then add perfumed magnesium carbonate and mix properly. Serve the powder and pack in to containers.

Evaluation

(i)   *Shade control and lighting :* Spread out powder on white paper and compare with the skin tone or undue tone.

(ii) *Dispersion of Color :* Spread powder on white paper and check with magnifying glass for homogeneous distribution of color. There should be no segregation or bleeding of color.

(iii) *Pay off :* Testing of adhesion with the puff. Puff press on powder, apply on skin. The powder should be pay off on skin completely, means good pay off property.

(iv) *Flow property :* Measured by angle of repose.

(v)   *Particle size :* Particle size is determined by microscopically or by sieve analysis. The particle size should be finely divided.

(v)   *Abrasiveness :* It is check by rubbing powder on smooth surface, and then check that surface microscopically.

(vi) *Limits of color :* Assay for color by analytical method.

Use : As anti-perspiring and soothing effect.

Exercise - 27

Object : To prepare and evaluate "Talcum Powder".

Formula :

Thymol	:	1%
Boric acid	:	10%
Zinc oxide	:	20%
Talcum	:	69%

Method : Mix all ingredients thoroughly in ascending order in the form of fine particles and then pack in to suitable containers.

Evaluation : Evaluate as earlier exercise.

Use : As foot deodorant, astringent effect, anti-perspirant, and disinfectant.

Exercise - 28

Object : To prepare and evaluate "Face Powder".

Formula :

Zinc oxide	:	5%
Rice starch	:	10%
Zinc stearate	:	5%
Talcum	:	80%
Coloring agent	:	q.s.
Perfume	:	q.s.

Method : Add perfume to rice starch and kept aside for few hours. Mix fine particles of all ingredients homogeneously. Finally, add perfume and mix well then pack in to jars or plastic bottles.

Evaluation : Evaluate as Exercise No. 26

Use : Used for masking the skin imperfection and to increase covering effect.

Exercise - 29

Object : To prepare and evaluate "Face Powder".

Formula :

Zinc stearate	:	15.0 gm
Zinc oxide	:	17.5 gm
Calcium carbonate	:	20.0 gm
Talc	:	47.0 gm
Color	:	0.2 gm
Perfume	:	0.3 gm

Method : Finely powdered all the ingredients. Add perfume with calcium carbonate and keep aside for some time. Mix color (lakes/organic or inorganic pigment iron oxide for yellow, red and brown color, ultramarine for green and blue color) with parts of talc properly. Mix colored powder and finely powdered ingredient thoroughly and lastly adds perfumed powder. Pass the powdered mixture through silk mesh or old washed nylon cloth and then pack.

Evaluation : Evaluate as earlier exercise.

Use : To hide skin blemishes.

Exercise - 30

Object : To prepare and pack "Compact Powder".

Formula :

	Titanium dioxide	:	4%
	Colloidal kaolin	:	16.5%
	Rice starch	:	4%
	Zinc stearate	:	6%
	Talcum	:	60%
	Magnesium carbonate	:	5%
	Colors	:	4%
	Perfume	:	0.5%
Binders	Mineral oil	:	2%
	Lanolin	:	3%
	Cetyl alcohol	:	4%
	Triethanolamine		
	Lauryl sulfate	:	1%
	Sodium alginate	:	1%
	Alcohol	:	4%
	Water	:	82.5%
	Glycerol	:	2%

Method : Binder preparation: -   Stir the solution of glycerol dry ethanolamine lauryl Sulphate in half of the water at (85°C) in to the melt of lanolin, mineral oil and cetyl alcohol (85°C). Damper the mucins with alcohol (sodium alginate), pours the remaining water (90°C) over them, and stirs until the solution is smooth.

Powder

Blend Preparation : Pours perfume oil over magnesium carbonate and leave for 24 hours. Then combine it with the other ingredient in a powder mixture, mix for about 2 hours, take a sample, grind it and check for color, uniformity and particle size. If every parameter is satisfactory, the powder itself will be ready for grinding. Mix 90 parts of powder with 10 parts of binder and prepare cakes by the wet or dry method.

Wet method : Basic materials, colors and binders are added in to a paste with water, pressed in to molds and slowly air-dried.

Dry method : Compacts are made by simple pressure of the dried mixture in special presses under strictly controlled condition.

Use : To hide blemishes of skin and protective.

Exercise - 31

Object : To prepare and pack "Compact Powder".

Formula :

(A) Powder Blend

Titanium dioxide	:	4%
Colloidal kaolin	:	16.5%
Rice starch	:	4.0%
Zinc stearate	:	6.0%
Talcum	:	60.0%
Magnesium carbonate	:	5.0%
Colors	:	4.0%
Perfume	:	0.5%

(B) Binder

Carboxymethylcellulose	:	1.0%
Low viscosity		
Sodium alginate	:	0.5%
Alcohol	:	2.0%
Water	:	96.3%
Methyl-p-hydroxy benzoate	:	0.2%

Method : Pour perfume oil over magnesium carbonate and leave for 24 hours. Then combined with other ingredients of powder mixture thoroughly. Pass through fine sieves. Separately prepare binder solution:- adding preservative in water and heat to 90°C and side by side carboxymethylcellulose and sodium alginate wetted by alcohol. To those wetted mixtures add hot water solution with stirring until they are completely dissolved. Mix 93 parts of powder blend with 7 parts of binder and press in to cakes.

Use :

1. It gives velvety peach like complexion.

2. It improves adherence of lanugo hairs resulting accentuation.

Exercise - 32

Object : To prepare and evaluate "Tooth Powder".

Formula :

Phenol	:	2.5 gm
Kiesulghur	:	57.5 gm
Calcium carbonate (heavy)	:	40.0 gm
Flavor	:	q.s.
Color	:	q.s.

Method : Flavor is sprayed or premixed with abrasive and polishing agents i.e., calcium carbonate and kiesulghur, and then mixed with bulk.

Evaluation

1. *Identification and evaluation of ingredient:* It is carried out by analytical method

2. *Abrasiveness:* Evaluate as in Exercise No. 26

3. *Particle size:* Evaluate as in Exercise No. 26

4. Cleansing property :

    (i) *In-vitro* : By change in reflection character of a lacquer cooling on a polyethylene film caused by brushing with a tooth powder.

    (ii) *In-vivo* : Teeth were brushed for 2 weeks and conditions of teeth were assessed before and after use with the help of photograph.

5. *Rheology :* Flow property by determining angle of repose, which should be < 30°.

6. *pH of the product* : Take the pH of 10% of the product in water, should have similar pH to tooth i.e., 7.0.

7. *Foaming character :* Product with equal amount of water and then shakes and study the nature of foaming.

    (i) *Stability of foam :* Observe the time for foam to be stable.

    (ii) *Washability :* Observe complete washing of foam when it is washed by water.

8. *Limit test for arsenic and lead :* Test is performed as given in official books.

Use : For cleaning the teeth and remove fresh plaque.

Exercise - 33

Object : To prepare and evaluate "Tooth Powder".

Formula :

Calcium carbonate	:	84.0 gm
Tricalcium phosphate	:	10.0 gm
Sodium lauryl sulphate	:	3.0 gm
Sodium perborate	:	2.0 gm
Saccharin sodium	:	1.0 gm
Flavor	:	q.s.
Color	:	q.s.

Method : Flavor is sprayed or premixed with calcium carbonate, tricalcium phosphate and then mixed with the bulk.

Evaluation : As given Exercise No. 32.

Use : As mouth freshener and teeth cleaner.

Exercise - 34

Object : To prepare and pack "Tooth Paste".

Formula :

Calcium carbonate	:	44.5 gm
Magnesium carbonate	:	1.0 gm
Magnesium hydroxide	:	3.0 gm
Sodium lauryl sulphate	:	1.0 gm
Cream tragacanth	:	1.0 gm
Glycerin	:	31.0 gm
Oil of peppermint	:	1.0 gm
Saccharine	:	0.1 gm
Water	:	18.4 gm
Preservative	:	q.s.

(P-hydroxy benzoate 0.15%)

(Propyl-P-hydroxy benzoate 0.02%)

Method : Firstly gum is mixed with humectant for proper dispersion. Other powdered ingredients are sifted together and added gradually to mucilaginous mixture with continuous gentle stirring. The aqueous media is mixed and stirred to get product. Flavors and detergent are added in last and then packed.

Use : For cleaning teeth and mouth freshener.

Exercise 35

Object : To prepare and pack "Denture Cleansers".

Formula :

Dental soap	:	16.0 gm
Calcium carbonate	:	80.0 gm
Glycerin	:	3.0 gm
Saccharin sodium	:	0.1 gm
Color	:	q.s.
Flavor	:	q.s.

Method : Firstly the soap and calcium carbonate are mixed along with glycerin. Other ingredients are then mixed with same water. These all are mixed together and made in to bars, by mechanical process.

Use : For removing plaque and calculus disposed on teeth.

Exercise - 36

Object : To prepare and evaluate "Hair Conditioner".

Formula :

Acetylated lanolin	:	3.5%
Cetyl monostearate (self emulsifying)	:	13.5%
Spermaceti	:	1.5%
Amerchol L-101	:	9.0%
Mineral oil (70 – viscosity)	:	8.5%
Glycerol	:	4.5%
Water	:	59.5%
Perfume, color, preservative	:	q.s.

Method : Melt the oil at about 85°C. Dissolve the water-soluble materials in the water. Mix the two phases at about 85°C and cool it and mix it slowly.

Evaluation : The following evaluations are carried out by following procedures as given in evaluation chapter:-

(i)   pH

(ii)   Viscosity

(iii) Strengthening property

(iv) Lustrous property

(v)   Cleansing efficiency

(vi) Smoothening and appearance

(vii) Time period - effects

Use : To provide glaze and shine hairs, to maintain healthy hairs.

Exercise - 37

Object : To prepare and evaluate "Hair Conditioners".

Formula :

Tagamine S-13	:	4%
Citric acid	:	1%
WSP – X250	:	10%
Water	:	85%
Preservative	:	q.s.
Color, perfume	:	q.s.

Method : Dissolve Tagamine S-13 (a emulsifier) in a part of water and heat it. Combine aqueous solution of citric acid and mix well. Then add WSP-X250 (a protein hydrolysate), color, preservative and perfume. While mixing cool and pack in to bottles.

Use :

1. Used as protein conditioners.

2. As instant conditioners.

Exercise - 38

Object : To prepare and pack "Lipsticks".

Formula :

Bees wax	:	15%
Ozokerite	:	10%
Carnauba wax	:	5%
Ceresin wax	:	4%
Lanolin absorption base	:	14%
Isopropyl myristate	:	10%
Diethyl sebacate	:	10%
Castor oil	:	15%
Eosin	:	2%
Color lakes	:	10%
Butylated hydroxy toluene	:	q.s.
Perfume	:	q.s.

Method : Bases are arranged accordingly to consistency with the hardest wax at the top to thinnest liquid at the bottom. Then melt the based from bottom to top and make liquid phase of base then incorporate color (10%).

Use : As coloring of lips.

Exercise 39

Object : To prepare and pack "Lipstick".

Formula :

Carnauba wax	:	10%
Bees wax	:	15%
Lanolin	:	5%
Cetyl alcohol	:	5%
Castor oil	:	65%
Staining dye	:	1%
Pigment	:	5%
Perfume	:	0.5%
Antioxidant	:	0.1%

Method : Melt the oils and waxes in a crucible with increasing melting point at 70°C – 75°C with stirring then add rest ingredient except perfume. Perfume is added in melted cool mixture at 42°C. Then fill in to mold.

Use : As decorative preparation.

Exercise - 40

Object : To prepare and pack "Eye Liner".

Formula :

Paraffin	:	29%
Carnauba	:	5%
Bees wax	:	21%
Petrolatum viscous	:	21%
Lanolin	:	9%
Cetyl alcohol	:	8%
Lamp black color	:	10%

Method : Melt all the oily material with increasing melting point. Add color in melted fats with stirring. Homogenize and fill in to mold.

Use : To accentuate the eye and finally apparent appearance.

Exercise - 41

Object : To prepare and pack "Liquid Soap".

Formula :

Fatty acid (as sodium salt)	:	78 – 80%
Glycerol	:	0 – 1%
Common salt	:	0.2 – 0.5%
Free alkali	:	0.03 – 0.05%
Resin	:	0 – 2 %
Super fatting agents	:	0 – 2%
Whitening, chelating agents	:	q.s.
Antioxidants & pigments		
Perfume	:	0.5 – 3%
Water	:	100%

Method : Dissolve all ingredients in to water thoroughly except perfume. After that complete dissolution add perfume homogeneously and fill in to containers.

Use : As washing the skin.

Exercise - 42

Object : To prepare and pack "Liquid Soap".

Formula :

Water	:	53.6%
Isopropyl alcohol	:	36.4%
Glycerol	:	1.5%
Hamamelis water	:	5%
Normolactol	:	0.5%
Rose	:	25

Method : Mix all ingredients thoroughly.

Use : As washing skin with protective action.

Exercise - 43

Object : To prepare and pack "Liquid Soap".

Formula :

Water	:	58.9%
Ethyl alcohol (96%)	:	28.4%
Propylene Glycol	:	6.7%
Boric acid	:	2.0%
Zinc pheno-sulphate	:	1.1%
Benzoic acid	:	2.1%
Menthol	:	0.1%
Perfume	:	0.7%

Method : Dissolve the solids in the mixture of propylene glycol and water. Stir in the solution of methanol and perfume oil in alcohol. Filter after a maturing period of about two weeks.

Use : To wash skin.

Exercise - 44

Object : To prepare and pack "Soap".

Formula :

Tallow	:	15%
Coconut oil	:	10%
Stearic acid	:	10%
Sodium hydroxide	:	5%
Potassium hydroxide	:	10%

Method : The soap prepared by the semi-boiled method of adding the sodium hydroxide to the mixture of tallow and coconut oil in a crutcher heated to 110 – 120°F, after which the potassium hydroxide is added, followed by the melted stearic acid. The crutcher is then heated to about 158°F and held until saponification is completed. Adjustment for free alkali or fatty acids is then made. The soap pour in to molds while fluid or can be chipped, dried, milled, plodded or pressed in to suitable cake shapes.

Use : To wash skin with prevention from dryness.

Exercise - 45

Object : To prepare and pack "Baby Powder".

Formula :

Talc	:	87.0 gm
Magnesium stearate	:	5.0 gm
Magnesium carbonate (light)	:	5.0 gm
Boric acid	:	2.5 gm
Perfume oil	:	0.5 gm

Method : Finely powder all materials. Add perfume oil with magnesium carbonate and keep it aside for some time. Mix talc with finely powdered ingredients thoroughly and lastly adds perfumed powder. Pass the powder mixture through silk mesh or old washed nylon cloth and then pack.

Use : As antiseptic, disinfectant powder.

Exercise - 46

Object : To prepare and pack "Baby Powder".

Formula :

Talc	:	97.25%
Olive oil	:	2.50%
Perfume	:	0.25%

Method : Mix all ingredients in fine powder thoroughly.

Use : For soothing effect.

Exercise - 47

Object : To prepare and pack "Liquid Soap".

Formula :

Coconut oil	:	18.0%
Castor oil	:	4.07%
Potassium hydroxide 85%	:	5.3%
Glycerol	:	4.0%
Perfume	:	0.2%
Water	:	68.0%
Borax	:	0.5%

Method : Dissolve potassium hydroxide solution in water to make 50% of solution and warm slightly. Mix both the oils and warm it to the temperature of alkali solution is added to oils in a thin jet under constant stirring. Add borax solution to the mixture give neutral pH. Allow cooling at room temperature and then adding glycerol. This liquid soap is stored for at least a week at room temperature. Then add perfume and mix well and filter then filled in to bottles.

Use : Use as soap shampoo.

Herbal Cosmetics

The biggest problem faced in making cosmetic products is shelf life. They do have to be made more often as they tend to spoil after a certain amount of time, but the quality of the product and the knowledge you are using only the best ingredients far outweighs the small inconvenience. Do not use your fingers, Use a small spatula or plastic knife or similar sterile utensil to lift out a small amount at a time when using the product.

By themselves, oils and waxes will remain stable. It is the introduction of the herbal infusion, or aloe gel, or unsterilized water that presents the problem of mold and bacteria. It is also possible to make or purchase extracts of the herbs you wish to include and use those in your products, rather than an infusion. Oils commonly used in cosmetic preparations are sweet almond, olive, safflower, peanut, corn, wheat germ, jojoba, and small amounts of vitamin E oil. Vitamin E can be purchased in gel caps which can then be pierced and the contents squeezed out. In the following recipes the ingredient lecithin refers to liquid lecithin. All lanolin used is anhydrous lanolin. Lanolin comes in liquid and anhydrous (water removed) forms. One other ingredient you will require is beeswax. It melts at 148°F, but the process goes more quickly if you first grate it. A hand held rotary grater with the large holes for grating makes short work of this. Other tools which you will need are a blender, or mini food processor, or similar item which is capable of making mayonnaise, since the process of combining oils and water is similar. You will also need a stainless steel or enamel double boiler. It is absolutely essential to melt the waxes and oils in the top portion of the double boiler over hot water in the bottom pan

This part will specially covers the method of preparation of various types of herbal cosmetic formulations.

Exercise - 48

Object : To prepare and pack "Lime complexion Lotion"

Formula :

Lime flowers	:	25 gm
Distilled water	:	250 ml
Sodium benzoate	:	1 ml

Method : Put the lime flowers in boiling water for an hour. Strain and let the mixture cool. Add sodium benzoate to it. Keep it under refrigeration and use it with the help of cotton buds.

Use : This is a very good complexion lotion Complexion lotions/sunscreen lotions for all skin types. Complexion lotions not only improve the colour of the skin but also protect it from the harmful effects of the sun by providing a screen between skin and the sunrays. Therefore they are generally known as sunscreen lotions.

Exercise - 49

Object : To prepare and pack "Lavender Complexion Lotion"

Formula :

Borax powder	:	7 gm
Rose water	:	250 ml
Olive oil	:	30 ml
Lavender ext.	:	125 ml

Method : Mix borax powder in rose water and add boiling oil to the mixture. Keep stirring, when cool, add lavender extract too. It can be kept under refrigeration for more than 2 months.

Use : Protect skin from sun burns. Before applying wash your skin properly.

Exercise - 50

Object : To prepare and pack "Almond Complexion Lotion"

Formula :

Almond Oil	:	15 ml
Cucumber/carrot juice	:	5 ml
Glycerine	:	10 ml
Liquid paraffin	:	5 ml
Cornflower ext.	:	5 ml

Method : Heat the almond oil and paraffin together and add all the other ingredients to it. Then cool it and fill into proper containers.

Use : Shake it well, apply it and let it remain till it dries. Rinse off with cold water preceded by luke warm water wash. It leaves the skin looking fairer and smoother.

Exercise - 51

Object : To prepare and pack "Sesame Complexion Lotion"

Formula :

Sesame oil	:	40 ml
Olive oil	:	10 ml
Almond oil	:	10 ml
Neem oil	:	Q.S.

Method : Mix all the oils together and properly filled into the glass bottles to protect it from light.

Use : Apply it on the face and neck. It is an exclusive tonic to protect the skin from scorching heat of sun or is a very effective measure to get rid of sun tanning.

Exercise - 52

Object : To prepare and pack "Brook Lime Complexion Lotion"

Formula :

Leaves/stems of brook lime	:	50 gm
Distilled water	:	500 ml
Sodium benzoate	:	2 ml

Method : Boil the water and put the brook lime leaves/stems in it. Leave it for an hour. Strain and let it cool. Now mix sodium benzoate in it. It can be kept under refrigeration for more than 2 months.

Use : Apply it on the face and neck with cotton. It removes the spots and blackheads.

Exercise - 53

Object : To prepare and pack "Pimple Removing Tomato Lotion"

Formula :

       Camphor lotion :   5 ml

       Tomato juice   :   5 ml

       Honey   :   5 ml

Method : Mix all the ingredients well and semi solid paste will be formed.

Use : Apply the paste on the face. Leave it on for 15 minutes. The wash off with lukewarm water followed by a cold water rinse. It is very good for removing spots caused by pimples.

Exercise - 54

Object : To prepare and pack "Pimple Removing Garlic Lotion"

Formula :

Multani mitti powder	:	14 gm
Honey	:	5 ml
Carrot Juice	:	5 ml
Garlic (paste)	:	1 ml

Method : Blend all these together and store properly the prepared paste.

Use : Apply this mask on the face for 20 minutes. After that wash off with lukewarm water. Never forget to give a cold water rinse because the pores which get opened by lukewarm water wash, get contracted if you rinse off with cold water.

Exercise - 55

Object : To prepare and pack "Pimple Removing Camphor Lotion"

Formula :

Glycerin	:	5 ml
Borax powder	:	7 gm
Distilled water	:	250 ml
Camphor lotion	:	1 ml

Method : Mix all these ingredients well and make a mixture of it, keep it into refrigerator.

Use : Apply this on the face and leave it to dry. When it is dry, wash off with lukewarm water. Finally rinse off with cold water. It removes the black scars.

Exercise - 56

Object : To prepare and pack "Lemon Astringent Lotion"

Formula :

Lemon juice	:	10 ml
Distilled water	:	240 ml
Tincture of benzoin	:	15 ml

Method : Mix all the ingredients together and keep it in cool place.

Use : Useful to cure acne. Apply it with a cotton pad.

Exercise - 57

Object : To prepare and pack "Cornflower Astringent Lotion"

Formula :

      Distilled water   :   250 ml

      Cornflower   :   100 gm

      Witch hazel   :   5 ml

Method : Boil the water and soak the corn flower in it. Strain the mixture and mix with hazel.

Use : Soaking the cotton pad in this mixture an then applyit on the desired places. Useful for acne prone skin.

Exercise - 58

Object : To prepare and pack "Rose Astringent Lotion"

Formula :

      Rose petals/roots   : 500 gm

      Distilled water   : 1.50 litres

      Sodium benzoate   : 3.5 gm

Method : Boil the water and soak the rose petals in it. Then mix sodium benzoate in the mixture.

Use : Apply it with cotton pads. It is very good for tightening the skin and removing the wrinkles.

Exercise - 59

Object : To prepare and pack "Lilly Astringent Lotion"

Formula :

Distilled water	:	2 litres
Lilly flower	:	500 gm
Sodium benzoate	:	3.5 gm

Method : Soak the lilly flower in boiling water for an hour. Then strain and mix sodium benzoate in it.

Use : Soak cotton buds in the mixture and apply it on the face. It leaves the skin fair and soft.

Exercise - 60

Object : To prepare and pack "Nutmeg Astringent Lotion"

Formula :

Honey	:	15 ml
Nutmeg powder	:	14 gm
Clove powder	:	7 gm
Grated lemon peels	:	28 gm
Brandy	:	30 ml
Rose water	:	60 ml
Orange flower extract	:	30 ml
Tincture of benzoin	:	1 ml

Method : Mix them thoroughly. Let it stand for 7 days, the store it in proper containers. It can be keep for more than 2 months if kept under refrigeration.

Use : Apply with cotton or by hand and leave it for15minutes. Make the skin firm and glowy.

Exercise - 61

Object : To prepare and pack "Peppermint Astringent Lotion"

Formula :

Calamine lotion	:	60 ml
Witch hazel extract	:	60 ml
Peppermint extract	:	30 ml
Vinegar (cider)	:	5 ml
Tincture of benzoin	:	15 ml

Method : Mix them thoroughly in mortar pestle and transfer it into bottles.

Use : Apply on the face for deep cleansing and opening of pores. Keep the remaining under refrigeration for further applications.

Exercise - 62

Object : To prepare and pack "Sandalwood Astringent Lotion"

Formula :

Sandalwood oil	:	120 ml
Sodium bicarbonate	:	5 gm
Almond oil	:	10 ml
Rose water	:	60 ml
Orange flower extract	:	60 ml
Honey	:	15 ml

Method : Mix all these ingredients well. Keep it under refrigeration so that you can preserve it for months.

Use : Reduce wrinkles and impart firmness to skin.

Exercise - 63

Object : To prepare and pack "Lemon Astringent Lotion"

Formula :

Sodium benzoate	:	7 gm
Rosemary powder	:	28 gm
Orange peels	:	14 gm
Lemon peels	:	28 gm
Mint leaves	:	30 leaves
Brandy	:	50 ml
Rose water	:	250 ml

Method : Soak orange peels, lemon peels and mint leaves in boiling rose water. Leave it so for an hour. Then strain and mix all the other ingredients to the mixture. Mix them thoroughly and keep under refrigeration into proper containers.

Use : Reduce wrinkles and impart firmness to skin.

Exercise - 64

Object : To prepare and pack "Witch Hazel Astringent Lotion"

Formula :

Rose water	:	250 ml
Witch hazel extract	:	30 ml
Tincture of benzoin	:	15 ml

Method : Mix them thoroughly. Keep it under refrigeration for further applications.

Use : Impart glow and firmness to skin. Apply on the face and neck at night.

Exercise - 65

Object : To prepare and pack "Grapefruit Skin Toning Lotion"

Formula :

Grapefruit (ripe)	:	100 gm
Yoghurt	:	250 gm
Sodium benzoate	:	3.5 gm

Method : Remove the skin of the grapefruit and cut it into small pieces. Put the pieces through the blender then mix with youghurt to make a paste. Refrigerate for an hour and add sodium benzoate, mix it properly and store.

Use : Smear over the face and neck. Leave for 30 minutes until you feel your pores tightening. Wash off with lukewarm water. It is very good for oily and sensitive skin

Exercise - 66

Object : To prepare and pack "Sunflower Skin Toning Lotion"

Formula :

Lanolin	:	250 ml
Sunflower oil	:	250 ml
Wheat germ oil	:	5 ml
Witch hazel extract	:	125 ml
Sodium benzoate	:	5 ml

Method : Melt lanolin in a pan over a low flame and stir in sunflower oil. Remove from the heat and stir in wheat germ oil and witch hazel with sodium benzoate. Transfer it into a bottle and refrigerate.

Use : Apply and massage a little into the face and neck at bed time. It is an effective tonic for dry skin. Wheat germ oil or vitamin E oil is very effective for dry skin. Apply it by dipping cotton bud in the oil. Rub a piece of potato over the face and neck and leave the juice for 15 minutes to dry on and then wash off. It is very effective for oily skin and can also be used for dry skin with a moisturiser.

Exercise - 67

Object : To prepare and pack "Cucumber Skin Soothing Preparation"

Formula :

Cucumber	:	100 gm
Yoghurt	:	100 gm

Method : Put the cucumber grind it through by blender and mix it with the yoghurt.

Use : Apply the paste on the face and neck. Leave to dry and then wash off with cold water. This is a good preparation for normal and sensitive skin.

Exercise - 68

Object : To prepare and pack "Witch Hazel Skin Soothing Preparation"

Formula :

Cucumber	:	100 gm
Honey	:	5 ml
Witch hazel extract	:	5 ml

Method : Grind the cucumber and mix honey and witch hazel to the pulp of cucumber. Keep in proper container at cool place.

Use : Apply on the face and neck, and leave it on for 20 minutes. When dry, wash off with cold water. This gives a luxurious touch to the dry skin.

Exercise - 69

Object : To prepare and pack "Almond Cleansing Cream"

Formula :

White beeswax	:	120 gm
Almond oil	:	500 ml
Rose water	:	250 ml
Borax powder	:	7 gm

Method : Heat the beeswax in a saucepan. When it is melted, add almond oil, rose water and borax powder. Mix them thoroughly and keep stirring till the mixture cools. It can be kept under refrigeration for a long time.

Exercise - 70

Object : To prepare and pack "Cucumber Cleansing Cream"

Formula :

Beeswax	:	30 gm
Spermaceti	:	30 gm
Olive oil	:	500 ml
Cucumber juice	:	125 ml
Sodium benzoate	:	5 ml

Method : Put a bowl in an open pot filled with boiling water. Pour spermaceti and beewax in the bowl. After they have melted, remove the bowl form the pot. Pour olive oil and cucumber juice. Keep stirring while the mixture is still warm and sodium benzoate.

Use : Protect the skin from the drying effects of cold wind.

Exercise - 71

Object : To prepare and pack "Lightweight Face & Body Cream"

Formula :

Coconut oil	:	43 ml
Sweet almond oil	:	31 ml
Vegetable glycerin	:	31 ml
Rosewater (or sterile water)	:	150 ml
Liquid lecithin	:	15 ml
Grated beeswax	:	7 gm
Tincture of Benzoin	:	9 drops

Method : Melt waxes, fats, liquid lecithin, in the top of a double boiler over simmering water. Watch that the mixture gets only warm enough to melt the contents. Beeswax should be grated for easiest melting. Make sure all is blended well and then remove from heat. Allow to cool about a minute. In a mixer bowl or lender, add the water, glycerin, the tincture of Benzoin. While blender or mixer is operating, slowly drizzle the warm melted oils and waxes into the water mixture. It will become thick. The longer you blend, the fluffier it will become. It will appear to be a little 'loose' at this point, but will continue to harden as it comes to room temperature. Pour into a suitable jar and allow to sit on the counter for 20 to 30 minutes, then cap and store in the refrigerator.

Use : As a moisturizer.

Exercise - 72

Object : To prepare and pack "Aloe Moisturizing Hand Cream"

Formula :

Rosewater	:	50 ml
Aloe gel	:	15 ml
Sweet almond oil	:	25 ml
Peanut oil	:	7 ml
Cocoa butter	:	7 gm
Olive oil	:	7 ml
Anhydrous lanolin	:	1 ml
Liquid lecithin	:	7 ml
Grated beeswax	:	3.5 gm
Vitamin E	:	16 mg
Tincture of Benzoin	:	6 drops

Method : Melt liquid lecithin, cocoa butter , in the top of a double boiler over simmering water. Watch that the mixture gets only warm enough to melt the contents. Beeswax should be grated for easiest melting. Make sure all is blended well and then remove from heat. Allow to cool about a minute. To this add the vitamin E if it is used. Make sure all is well combined. Place aloe gel in blender and whip for a bit. Add rosewater to aloe and blend. Stir tincture of benzoin (or grapeseed extract, if desired) and vitamin E into the warm oils. With blender running, slowly drizzle the oils into the aloe-water mix. Put up into suitable containers and store in refrigerator. Shelf life is about one month. This cream is designed for work-worn hands in need of soothing repair.

Use : Very good moisturizer fro dry skin provides softness and removes itching.

Exercise - 73

Object : To prepare and pack "Hand Lotion"

Formula :

Coconut oil	:	50 ml
Sweet almond oil	:	75 ml
Vegetable glycerin	:	3 oz
Liquid lecithin	:	7 gm
Grated beeswax	:	3.5 gm
Tincture of benzoin	:	8 drops

Method : Melt wax and oils in top of double boiler. Place glycerin in bottom of bowl or blender. Turn on machine and begin to drizzle the oil mix into the glycerin per procedure mentioned above.

Exercise - 74

Object : To prepare and pack "Rich Face and Hand Cream "

Formula :

Rosewater	:	50 ml
Vegetable glycerin	:	7 ml
Sweet almond oil	:	25 ml
Coconut oil	:	7 ml
Peanut oil	:	7 ml
Anhydrous lanolin	:	1 ml
Liquid lecithin	:	7 ml
Cocoa butter	:	7 gm
Grated beeswax	:	3.5 gm.
Vitamin E	:	16 mg

Method : Melt waxes, fats, liquid lecithin, cocoa butter and honey in the top of a double boiler over simmering water. Watch that the mixture gets only warm enough to melt the contents. Beeswax should be grated for easiest melting. Make sure all is blended well and then remove from heat. Allow to cool about a minute. Make sure all is well combined. Add glycerin and extract to rosewater and blend. While blender is running, drizzle in the combined melted waxes and oils to which the vitamin E has been added. When well blended, transfer to a suitable container. Cover and refrigerate.

Use : Nourishes the skin

Bibliography

1. Farage MA, Miller KW, Elsner P et al., (2008): Intrinsic and extrinsic factors in skin ageing: A review. *Int J Cosmet Sci* **30(2)**: 87-95.

2. Dinkova-Kostova AT, Talalay P (2008): Direct and indirect antioxidant properties of inducers of cytoprotective proteins. *Mol Nutr Food Res* **52(1)**:S128-S136.

3. Liu H, Dinkova-Kostova AT, Talalay P (2008): Coordinate regulation of enzyme markers for inflammation and for protection against oxidants and electrophiles. *Proc Natl Acad Sci USA* **105(41)**: 15926-15931.

4. Khan N, Mukhtar H (2008): Multitargeted therapy of cancer by green tea polyphenols. *Cancer Lett.* **269(2)**: 269-280.

5. Heber D (2008): Multitargeted therapy of cancer by ellagitannins. *Cancer Lett.* **269(2)**: 262-268.

6. Nandakumar V, Singh T, Katiyar SK (2008): Multi-targeted prevention and therapy of cancer by proanthocyanidins. *Cancer Lett.* **269(2)**: 378-387.

7. Ruiz PA, Braune A, Hölzlwimmer G et al., (2007): Quercetin inhibits TNF-induced NF-kappaB transcription factor recruitment to proinflammatory gene promoters in murine intestinal epithelial cells. *J Nutr* **137(5)**: 1208-1215.

8. Yang CS, Fang M, Lambert JD, et al., (2008): Reversal of hypomethylation and reactivation of genes by dietary polyphenolic compounds. *Nutr. Rev* **66(1)**: S18-S20.

9. Dinarello CA (2006): Inhibitors of histone deacetylases as anti-inflammatory drugs. *Ernst Schering Res Found Workshop* **56**:45-60.

10. Said R (2011): Inhibitors of serine proteinases, matrix metalloproteinases and histone deacetylases: Thermorubin, COL-308, myricetin, and tel-limagrandin. Paper presented at the URECA Celebration, Stony Brook University.

11. F. Afaq and H. Mukhtar (2002). Photochemoprevention by botanical antioxidants, Skin Pharmacol. *Appl. Skin Physiol.* **15(5):** 297–306.

12. S. F'guyer, F. Afaq, and H. Mukhtar (2003). Photochemoprevention of skin cancer by botanical agents. *Photo-dermatol. Photoimmunol. Photomed.***19(2):** 56–72

13. S. Saraf and C. D. Kaur (2010). Phytoconstituents as photoprotective novel cosmetic formulations, *Pharmacog. Rev.* **4(7):** 1–11.

14. C. Deep and S. Saraf (2009). Herbal photoprotective formulations and their evaluation. *Open Nat. Prod. J.* **2:** 71–76.

15. M. S. Ashawat, S. Saraf, and S. Saraf (2007). Biochemical and histopathological studies of herbal cream against UV radiation induced damage. *Trends Med. Res.* **2(3):** 135–141.

16. C. Deep and S. Saraf (2008). Novel approaches in herbal cosmetics. *J. Cosmet. Dermatol.* **7(2):** 89–95.

17. S. Mathew and T. E. Abraham (2006). Studies on the antioxidant activities of cinnamon (Cinnamomum verum) bark extracts through various in vitro models, *Food Chem.* **94(4):** 520–528.

18. M. S. Ashawat, S. Saraf, and S. Saraf (2008). Preparation and characterization of herbal creams for improvement of skin viscoelastic properties. *Int. J. Cosmet. Sci.* **30(3):** 183–193.

19. M. S. Ashawat, S. Saraf, and S. Saraf (2007). *In vitro* antioxidant activity of ethanolic extracts of Centella asiatica, Punica granatum, Glycyrrhiza glabraand, Areca catechu. *Res. J. Med. Plants.* **1(1):** 13–16.

20. F. Pittella, R. C. Dutra, D. D. Junior, et al., (2009). Antioxidant and cytotoxic activities of Centella asiatica (L) Urb. *Int. J. Mol. Sci.* **10(9):** 3713–3721.

21. R. Morisset, N. G. Cote, J. C. Panisset, et al., (1987). Evaluation of the healing activity of hydrocotyle tincture in the treatment of wounds. *Phytotherapy Res.* **1(3):** 117–121.

22. K. E. Siddig, H. P. M. Gunasena, B. A. Prasad, et al., (2006). Tamarind, *Tamarindus indica* L. Southampton Centre for Underutilised Crops. 26–32.

23. F. Martinello, S. M. Soares, J. J. Franco, et al., (2006). Hypolipemic and antioxidant activities from Tamarin-dus indica L. pulp fruit extract in hypercholesterolemic hamsters, *Food Chem. Toxicol.* **44(6):** 810–818.

24. B. J. Boucher and N. Mannan (2002). Areca nut symposium: Metabolic effects of the consumption of *Areca catechu*. *Addiction Biol.* **7(1):** 103–110.

25. A.K. Pandey and A. R. Chowdhury (2003). Volatile constituents of the rhizome oil of *Curcuma caesia* Roxb from central India. *Flavour Fragr. J.* **18(5):** 463–465.

26. D. K. Arulmozhi, N. Sridhar, A. Veeranjaneyulu, et al., (2007). Preliminary mechanistic studies on the smooth muscle relaxant effect of hydro alcoholic extract of Curcuma caesia. *J. Herbal Pharmacother.* **6(3-4):** 117–124.

27. Agro-Techniques of Selected Medicinal Plants (2008). Volume 1, (National Medicinal Plants Board, Department of AYUSH, Ministry of Health and Family Welfare; Government of India.) 73–74.

28. T. Forster and H. Tesmann (1991). Phase inversion emulsification. *Cosmet. Toiletr.* **11:** 106.

29. Methods of Testing for Safety Evaluation of Cosmetics, Indian Standard Bureau ARE 4011 (1997).

30. B. A. Louise (1998). Cosmetic Claim Substantiation (Marcel Dekker, New York). Vol. **18:** 97–99.

31. Indian Standard Bureau IS: 11648, 5.2 (1999).

32. J. S. Mansur, M. N. R. Breder, M. C. A. Mansur, and R. D. Azulay (1986). Determinação Do Fator De Proteção Solar Por Espectrofotometria. *An. Bras. Dermatol.* **61:** 121–124.

33. R. M. Sayre, P. P. Agin, G. J. Levee, and E. Marlowe (1979). Comparison of *in vivo* and *in vitro* testing of sun screening formulas. *Photochem. Photobiol.* **29:** 559–566.

34. C. D. Kaur and S. Saraf (2010). *In vitro* SPF determination of herbal oils used in cosmetics. *Pharmacog. Res.* **2(1):** 22–25.

35. Indian Standard Bureau IS: 4011; 4.3.1.3 (1997).

36. E. Yilmaz and H. Borcher (2006). Effect of lipid-containing positively charged nanoemulsions on skin hydration, elasticity and erythema: An *in vivo* study. *Int. J. Pharm.* **307(2):** 232–238.

37. S. Y. Pande and R. Misri (2005). Sebumeter, *Ind. J. Dermatol. Venereol.Leprol.* **71(6):** 444–446.

38. C. Edwards (1995). The Mexameter MX 16 TM in Bioengineering of the Skin: Methods and Instrumentation (CRC Press, Boca Raton, FL).

39. S. Kapoor and S. Saraf (2009). Age dependent studies as various skin parameters using cutometer. *Ind. J. Pharm. Educ. Res.* **43(4):** 338–345.

40. H. A. Liberman, M. M. Rieger, and G. S. Banker (1989). Pharmaceutical Dosage Form: Disperse Systems (Marcel Dekker, New York) Vol. **3:** 594.

41. R. M. Baird. "Microbiological Contamination of Manufactured Products: Official and Unofficial Limits," in Microbial Quality Assurance in Cosmetics, Toiletries and Non-Sterile Pharmaceuticals, 2nd Ed., R. M.

42. Baird and S. F. Bloomfield (1996). Eds. (Taylor and Francis, UK) pp. 235–251.

43. M. E. M. Braga, P. F. Leal, J. E. Carvalho and M. A. A. Meireles (2003). Comparison of yield, composition, and antioxidant activity of turmeric (*Curcuma longa* L.) extracts obtained using various techniques. *J. Agric. Food Chem.* **51(22):** 6604–6611.

44. M. Gallo, R. Ferracane, G. Graziani, A. Ritieni, and V. Fogliano (2010). Microwave assisted extraction of phenolic compounds from four different spices. *Molecules* **15(9):** 6365–6374.

45. Aburjai T, Natsheh FM (2003). Plants used in cosmetics. *Phytother Res.* **17(9):** 987–1000.

Model Questions

1. What are the functions of skin?

2. What are the functions of hair?

3. Define cosmetic according to FDA

4. What is the acid mantle?

5. What is the role of stratum corneum in skin?

6. Give composition of stratum corneum.

7. What are wrinkles?

8. What are the factors responsible for colour of the skin?

9. What is the composition of hairs?

10. Describe various parts of hairs?

11. Longitudinal cells present in which part of the hairs.

12. Where is keratohyaline present in hair?

13. What is melanin?

14. In which part of hair Splitting occurs?

15. Life span of body hairs ——————————————

16. Growth rate of body hairs ——————————————

17. Density of hairs ——————————————

18. Papilla is present in ———————— with hair part

19. Wrinkle on skin is due to ——————————————

20. How elasticity of skin is maintained.

21. What is the role of semi gel matrix in skin?

22. Where is collagen bundles found in skin

23. What is the function of papillary bodies

24. Luster of skin is due to ——————————————————

25. What is lanugo hair?

26. What is skin tanning?

27. How will you classify the facial preparations?

28. What are the face packs?

29. What is eye liner?

30. What is face mask?

31. What are the ideal characteristics of face mask?

32. Discoloration, bleeding and granule formation of oil and water in the formulation of cold cream prevent by ——————————

33. What is vanishing cream?

34. Vanishing cream is ———————————— emulsion.

35. What is light vanishing cream?

36. What is heavy vanishing cream?

37. What is cleansing cream?

38. After shave lotions contains ———————— by volume of alcohol.

39. Classify various types of shampoo.

40. Talcum powders are the protective preparations against ————

41. The ability of cleaning to the face ——————————

42. What is bloom?

43. What are dentifrices?

44. Abrasives are agent, which remove ——————————-

45. What is the composition of denture cleansers?

46. What are the application of protective creams and gels?

47. What are the physical parameters of the evaluation of facial cosmetics?

48. What do you mean by the esthetic evaluation?

49. How will you perform bloom test?

50. What are the methods for determining the angle of repose?

51. How will you determine the degree of luster?

52. How will you evaluate the hair conditioners?

53. What are the physical evaluation parameters of herbal cosmetics?

54. Irritation test carried out by applying product on the skin for ——————— minutes.

55. What is bleeding test?

56. What do you mean by spreadability and pourability?

57. How will you evaluate the preservatives used in cosmetics?

58. What do you mean by the excipients?

59. What are the ideal characteristics of ideal Excipients?

60. What are selection parameters of excipient in cosmetic formulations?

61. Cold cream used as ———————————————————-

62. What is the main problem associated with the preparation of herbal ——————————————— cosmetics.

63. Aloe vera containing creams generally used for ______________ which effect.

64. Cucumber juice is famous for which cosmetic effect?

65. Benzoic acid is added as ——————————— in cosmetic preparation.

66. Name some herbal preparations that are used as complexation cream.

67. Name some pimple reducing cream and astringent cream.

68. What are the beneficial effects of herbal astringent lotion?

69. What are the evaluation parameters for herbal cosmetics?

70. Write the method to prepare Rich Face and Hand Cream.

Index

www.ingramcontent.com/pod-product-compliance
Lightning Source LLC
LaVergne TN
LVHW021255210726
843527LV00003B/193